PSYCHOPHARMACOLOGY CASE STUDIES

Psychopharmacology Case Studies

Second Edition

DAVID S. JANOWSKY, MD
Professor and Chairman, Department of Psychiatry
University of North Carolina School of Medicine
Chapel Hill, North Carolina

DOMINICK ADDARIO, MD
Assistant Clinical Professor of Psychiatry
University of California, San Diego, School of Medicine
La Jolla, California

S. CRAIG RISCH, MD
Associate Professor of Psychiatry
University of California, San Diego, School of Medicine
La Jolla, California

THE GUILFORD PRESS
New York London

A Division of Guilford Publications, Inc.
200 Park Avenue South, New York, N.Y. 10003

Printed in the United States of America

Last digit is print number: 9 8 7 6 5 4 3 2 1

Library of Congress Cataloging-in-Publication Data

Janowsky, David S. (David Steffan), 1939–
Psychopharmacology case studies.

Includes bibliographies and index.
1. Psychopharmacology—Case studies. 2. Mental illness—Chemotherapy—Case studies. I. Addario, Dominick, 1944– . II. Risch, Samuel Craig. III. Title. [DNLM: 1. Mental Disorders—drug therapy—case studies. 2. Psychopharmacology—case studies. WM 402 J34p]
RC483.J36 1987 616.89'18 86-27049
ISBN 0-89862-687-0
ISBN 0-89862-921-7 (paperback)

INTRODUCTION

In this book we have presented a series of case studies which we believe outline current psychopharmacologic issues, dilemmas, or both. We have focused on cases that illustrate issues important in the treatment of affective disorders, schizophrenia, and neurotic disorders, as well as problems of children and the aged. In addition, we have included cases that illustrate the psychologic complications of general medical drug use. As a style of teaching we have selected the presentation of a case, followed by questions, a discussion, answers, and references, so as to make the issues considered more relevant and easy to remember.

We have tried to design this book to be useful as a teaching tool for psychiatrists, primary-care physicians, medical students, psychologists, psychiatric nurses, and other psychopathology-oriented professionals. An alternative use for our book is as an aid in preparing for professional specialty board examinations.

We have crafted our cases, questions, and answers to reflect issues, questions, and controversies presented to us in the context of university teaching rounds, and a variety of continuing-medical-education courses about which we have been repeatedly asked over the years by medical students, psychiatric residents, other physicians, and nurses.

The answers we consider "correct" represent a synthesis of opinions, derived from our collective clinical and academic experience, as well as from the references cited. They represent our best evaluation of the "state of the art" in the field of psychopharmacology. However, since we have attempted to present controversial issues and problems, we acknowledge that not all experts would agree with our opinions. Thus, most of all, we feel that in the field of psychopharmacology there are few absolutes. What is this year's dogma is next year's passé information. Therefore, it is hoped that as much as facilitating the acquisition of factual knowledge, this book will help its readers to orient themselves to the major issues and ambiguities that exist in the field of clinical psychopharmacology, and serve as a relevant basis for further learning.

David S. Janowsky, MD

CONTENTS

SECTION I: SCHIZOPHRENIC DISORDERS

1. Use of Antipsychotic Drugs in a Patient with Acute Schizophreniform Disorder 1
2. Utilization of Fluphenazine Enanthate in a Chronic Schizophrenic Patient 4
3. Rapid Tranquilization of a Patient with Acute Psychotic Symptoms 6
4. Treatment of a Chronically Relapsing Schizophrenic Patient 10
5. Side Effects of Antipsychotic Drugs in a Medication-Sensitive Patient 13
6. Maintenance Antipsychotic Drug Therapy 17
7. Tardive Dyskinesia in a Chronic Schizophrenic Patient 24
8. Antipsychotic-Drug-Induced Extrapyramidal Symptoms in a 28-Year-Old Woman 29
9. The Need for Antipsychotic Drug Maintenance in a Young Woman with Tardive Dyskinesia 32
10. Neuroleptic-Withdrawal-Induced Psychotic and Movement Disorders in a Schizophrenic Patient 37
11. Indications for Specific Antipsychotic Drugs in an Elderly Patient 40
12. Development of Tardive Dyskinesia in an Elderly Patient 43
13. Use of Reserpine in a Chronic Schizophrenic Patient 47
14. Tapering of Antipsychotic Drugs in a Relapse-Sensitive Patient 51

SECTION II: AFFECTIVE DISORDERS

15. Treatment of Unipolar Depression 53
16. Treatment of a Case of Depression with Imipramine 57

17. Differentiation of Dementia versus Pseudo-Dementia 61
18. Treatment of a Case of Resistant Depression 67
19. Antidepressant-Induced Side Effects 72
20. Use of Newer Antidepressants 75
21. Treatment of a Case of Mania with Lithium and Other Antimanic Drugs 78
22. Maintenance Drug Therapy in a Patient with Affective Disorder 83
23. Maintenance Therapy with Lithium Carbonate 91
24. Treatment of a Manic Patient with Carbamazepine 95
25. Lithium Carbonate as an Antidepressant 98
26. Treatment of Schizophreniform Disorder 99
27. Diagnosis and Treatment of Acute Mania 104
28. Prophylactic Lithium Carbonate Treatment 106
29. Electroconvulsive Therapy in an Elderly Patient 108
30. Treatment of Premenstrual Tension 113
31. Treatment of Depression in an Elderly Woman 115
32. Utilization of Antidepressants in the Elderly 119
33. Treatment of Mania in the Elderly 123
34. Interaction of Imipramine and Guanethidine 126
35. Combination Monoamine Oxidase Inhibitor–Tricyclic Antidepressant Therapy 128
36. Antidepressant Treatment in a Hemodialysis Patient 133
37. Diagnosis and Treatment of Mania in an Elderly Woman 138
38. Premenstrual Syndrome in a 35-Year-Old Woman 144

SECTION III: NEUROTIC DISORDERS

39. Treatment of Situational Anxiety 147
40. Treatment of Recurrent Panic Attacks 151
41. Treatment of Anxiety with Antianxiety Agents 155
42. Treatment of Anxiety with Propranolol 158
43. Evaluation and Treatment of Insomnia 161
44. Chronic Insomnia and Its Treatment 165

SECTION IV: ORGANIC BRAIN SYNDROME

45. Treatment of Acute-Onset Organic Brain Syndrome 169
46. Confusion in an Elderly Man 173

SECTION V: DRUG AND ALCOHOL ABUSE

47. Diazepam (Valium) Dependence 175
48. Sedative–Hypnotic Overdose 177
49. Drug Treatment of the Alcoholic 184
50. Withdrawal from Diazepam 191
51. Treatment of Wernicke–Korsakoff Syndrome 194
52. Heroin Detoxification in a Young Woman 197
53. Methadone Maintenance Therapy 201
54. Treatment of Pain in a Terminally Ill Patient 207
55. Treatment of an Adverse Lysergic Acid Diethylamide (LSD) Reaction 212
56. Sedative–Hypnotic Detoxification 213

SECTION VI: DISORDERS OF CHILDHOOD

57. Treatment of Enuresis 216
58. Treatment of Gilles de la Tourette Syndrome 221
59. Treatment of Hyperkinetic Child Syndrome 226

SECTION VII: IATROGENIC PSYCHOLOGIC DISORDERS

60. Depression Associated with Oral Contraceptives 234
61. Tricyclic-Antidepressant-Induced Central Anticholinergic Syndrome 237
62. Antihypertensive-Induced Depression 239
63. Psychosis following L-Dopa Therapy 242
64. Central Anticholinergic Syndrome following Ingestion of an Over-the-Counter Sleeping Preparation 248

Index 253

PSYCHOPHARMACOLOGY CASE STUDIES

SECTION I
SCHIZOPHRENIC DISORDERS

CASE 1: USE OF ANTIPSYCHOTIC DRUGS IN A PATIENT WITH ACUTE SCHIZOPHRENIFORM DISORDER

A 32-year-old white lawyer, who has successfully practiced law for 6 years, is married with two young sons and many close friends, and who is a popular Cub Scout leader, returns home from work to find his wife in bed with his best friend. Initially, he expresses much depression and anger, but within 2 days begins to speak of fusing with God, dispensing peace on Earth, and a need to fight the "giant conspiracy." He hears voices calling his name and saying "love, love, love." His affect becomes flat and he speaks slowly and distinctly. His sleep is not disturbed. He is admitted to a hospital where he is treated with perphenazine 40 mg per day. He improves rapidly. Within 4 days he begins conjoint therapy with his wife. He returns to work within 5 days of the onset of his initial symptoms.

1. It is quite possible that:
   A. The use of perphenazine may have been superfluous
   B. The perphenazine dose was two times that needed
   C. The psychiatric symptoms would probably have remitted spontaneously after a few days
   D. A and C
   E. None of the above
2. The patient probably has a diagnosis of:
   A. Acute schizophreniform disorder
   B. Acute paranoid disorder
   C. Bipolar disorder, manic
   D. Major depression

3. If antipsychotic medications are used, this patient should be maintained on antipsychotic agents for approximately:
   A. Two weeks to 1 month
   B. One to 2 years
   C. The rest of his life
4. The patient's chances of relapse, if antipsychotic medications are withdrawn, are:
   A. Rather likely
   B. Rather unlikely
   C. Certain
   D. Impossible

Case Continued: The patient is maintained on perphenazine for a period of 2 weeks, after which the drug is discontinued over a 2-day period. At his 2-month follow-up, the patient is doing well, and is without psychotic symptoms.

5. It is likely that:
   A. The perphenazine is still exerting its effect, since phenothiazine metabolites remain in the urine for many months after the perphenazine is discontinued
   B. The continuing remission is not directly related to a drug effect
6. In a patient with a good premorbid history, complete remission of symptoms, and no prior psychotic episodes, it is best to:
   A. Use maintenance antipsychotic medications
   B. Follow the patient closely for relapse and withhold maintenance antipsychotic medications
   C. Not start antipsychotic medications again if symptoms return
7. The dangers of giving a maintenance antipsychotic medication are:
   A. Tardive dyskinesia
   B. Reinforcement of the "sick" patient role
   C. A slight decrease in coordination and alertness
   D. All of the above
   E. None of the above

Discussion

The patient described above represents a common psychopharmacologic dilemma. A patient with no history of psychotic illness has an acute psychotic reaction following severe emotional stress. The dilemma is whether or not to start, and to continue, antipsychotic medications. Generally in such cases, antipsychotic medications are started too soon and continued too long. Many of these cases will remit spontaneously within a few days without antipsychotic medications. Return of symptoms may or may not occur with a recurrence of stress. Although differences of opinion exist on this matter, the authors believe it best to observe such an acutely psychotic patient with a good premorbid adjustment for several days without giving drugs, allowing the patient the possibility of integrating spontaneously and using his psychotic symptoms for growth. Whether to use long-term maintenance antipsychotic agents in such a case is more clear-cut. They should be avoided unless repeated episodes occur, since the risk of tardive dyskinesia, reinforcement of the "sick" patient role, and some mild decreases in coordination and alertness occur with chronic antipsychotic drug use. The prognosis in a patient such as is described above is quite good, and another such psychotic reaction may not occur again, or may not recur for many years. Too many patients are condemned to remaining on antipsychotic medications when such drugs are not indicated. Careful clinic monitoring can be substituted for chronic drug therapy.

Answers

1. (D)
2. (A)
3. (A)
4. (B)
5. (B)
6. (B)
7. (D)

References

1. Hollister, L. E.: Antipsychotic medications and the treatment of schizophrenia. In: *Psychopharmacology: From Theory to Practice* (eds.: J. D. Barchas, P. A. Berger, R. D. Ciaranello, and G. R. Elliott). Oxford University Press, New York, 1977, p. 121.
2. Hogarty, G. E. and Ulrich, R. F.: Temporal effects of drug and placebo in delaying relapse in schizophrenic outpatients. *Archives of General Psychiatry*, 34: 297–301, 1977.
3. Gardos, G. and Cole, J. O.: Maintenance antipsychotic therapy: Is the cure worse than the disease? *American Journal of Psychiatry*, 133: 32–36, 1977.

4. Kessler, K. A. and Waletzky, J. P.: Clinical use of the antipsychotics. *American Journal of Psychiatry*, 138: 202–209, 1981.
5. Linden, R. and Davis, J.: High- versus low-dose neuroleptics. *Psychiatric Annals*, 12: 769–781, 1982.
6. Donlon, P. and Tupin, J.: Overview: Efficacy and safety of rapid neuroleptization. *American Journal of Psychiatry*, 136: 273–278, 1979.
7. Tune, L., Creese, I., Depaulo, J. R., *et al.*: Clinical state and serum neuroleptic levels measured by radioreceptor assay in schizophrenia. *American Journal of Psychiatry*, 137: 187–190, 1980.
8. Brown, W., Laughren, T., Chisholm, E., and Williams, B. W.: Low serum neuroleptic levels predict relapse in schizophrenic patients. *Archives of General Psychiatry*, 39: 998–1000, 1982.

CASE 2: UTILIZATION OF FLUPHENAZINE ENANTHATE IN A CHRONIC SCHIZOPHRENIC PATIENT

A 45-year-old male chronic schizophrenic has a history of recurrent delusions of persecution and ideas of reference, as well as auditory persecutory hallucinations. He has a history of 19 inpatient psychiatric admissions. He generally will keep outpatient appointments, but forgets to take his antipsychotic medications. He usually relapses within 2 weeks of discontinuing his antipsychotic medications. While in the hospital, he has an alleviation of his psychotic symptoms when he receives 20 mg per day of fluphenazine hydrochloride (Prolixin) orally.

1. A reasonable treatment consists of:
   A. Switching the patient to chlorpromazine
   B. Placing the patient on a regimen of fluphenazine enanthate every 2 weeks
   C. Obtaining a conservatorship and placing the patient in a chronic-care facility
2. Fluphenazine enanthate:
   A. Is often effective in terminating the "revolving door" syndrome
   B. Should be given at three times the usual daily dose every 2 weeks
   C. Is given by i.m. injection
   D. Is indicated in patients in whom drug compliance is a problem
   E. All of the above
3. Prolixin enanthate is most effective when:

A. It is given at the request of the patient (when the patient feels he needs the drug)
B. It is given on a regular basis by a physician

4. In switching a patient from oral fluphenazine hydrochloride to fluphenazine enanthate:
   A. It is wise to taper the oral drug over a period of 4 to 6 days after the first injection of fluphenazine enanthate
   B. It is wise to abruptly discontinue the fluphenazine hydrochloride just after injection of fluphenazine enanthate
   C. The same dose as was given by mouth should be given every 2 weeks as the enanthate

Discussion

The development of fluphenazine enanthate appears to be a major step forward in the effective treatment of chronic schizophrenic patients who relapse due to a lack of drug compliance. Fluphenazine enanthate is a long acting, injectable form of fluphenazine which is effective for 1½ to 3 weeks. Many patients who would normally discontinue their medications remain on twice monthly fluphenazine injections and no longer relapse. Fluphenazine enanthate has been found to be most effective when the frequency and dosage of the drug are determined by the patient's physician, rather than by the patient. Generally, fluphenazine enanthate, given in a dose of approximately three times the daily oral dose, will effectively convert a patient from the oral to the intramuscular, long-acting form of the drug. Since it may initially take 3 to 6 days for i.m. fluphenazine enanthate to reach effective blood levels, it is wise to taper the oral fluphenazine dose over 3 to 6 days, following the first i.m. fluphenazine enanthate injection. Fluphenazine decanoate has also been developed, and is as long acting and effective as fluphenazine enanthate, and may have fewer side effects.

Answers

1. (B)
2. (E)
3. (B)
4. (A)

References

1. Ayd, F. J.: The depot fluphenazines: A reappraisal after ten years clinical experience. *American Journal of Psychiatry*, 132: 493, 1975.
2. Van Putten, T., Crumpton, E., and Yale, C.: Drug refusal in schizophrenia and the wish to be crazy. *Archives of General Psychiatry*, 33: 1443–1446, 1976.
3. Dysken, M., Javaid, J., Chang, S., *et al.*: Fluphenazine, pharmacokinetics and therapeutic response. *Psychopharmacology*, 73: 205–210, 1981.
4. Hollister, L. E. and Kim D. Y.: Intensive treatment with haloperidol of treatment-resistant chronic schizophrenic patients. *American Journal of Psychiatry*, 139: 1466–1473, 1982.
5. Lehmann, C. R., Ereshefsky, L., Saklad, S. R., and Mings, T. E.: Very high dose loxapine in refactory schizophrenic patients. *American Journal of Psychiatry*, 138(9): 1212–1214, 1981.
6. Grunhaus, L., Sancovici, S., and Ramon, R.: Neuroleptic melignant syndrome due to depot fluphenazine. *Journal of Clinical Psychiatry*, 40: 99–100, 1979.
7. Craig, T. J. and Lin, S. P.: Mortality among psychiatric inpatients. *Archives of General Psychiatry*, 38: 935–938, 1981.

CASE 3: RAPID TRANQUILIZATION OF A PATIENT WITH ACUTE PSYCHOTIC SYMPTOMS

Mr. N. is a 33-year-old unmarried white male who arrived at the emergency room of the university hospital complaining that spirits from God were controlling his mind. He was also noted to be hallucinating, hearing voices chanting, and hearing God telling him to sacrifice his left hand and his left eye. The patient's affect was very flattened, and he spoke with an obvious loosening of associations. He also demonstrated mild to moderate agitation. His history, as related by his sister, who accompanied him to the hospital, revealed that since age 25 he had had multiple psychiatric admissions, lasting from 1 to 3 months. He was unemployed but had worked intermittently as a waiter between episodes of psychosis. He was described as having been shy and withdrawn since childhood, with no current friends. His previous psychotic episodes generally were similar to the current one, and normally were preceded by the patient discontinuing his prescribed antipsychotic drugs. Two weeks prior to the current episode, the patient had moved out of his board and care facility and begun living in a low-cost hotel. He had stopped taking his haloperidol 2 weeks prior to admission.

1. The most likely diagnosis for this patient is:
   A. Catatonic schizophrenia
   B. Paranoid schizophrenia
   C. Bipolar disorder, manic type
   D. Transvestism
2. The most appropriate disposition for this patient is:
   A. Referral for outpatient psychotherapy and psychopharmacology
   B. Administration of 100 mg chlorpromazine immediately, with a return for re-evaluation the next day
   C. Immediate psychiatric hospitalization
   D. Referral to a psychiatric self-help group

Discussion

The patient was immediately admitted to the psychiatric inpatient unit. His mental status on admission was as described above. A physical examination was normal, and laboratory tests, including a chemistry panel, complete blood count, and urinalysis were also normal. Since the patient had heard voices telling him to mutilate his hand and eye, it was decided that a rapid neuroleptization protocol was indicated, and that the patient be put on one-to-one observation.

3. For rapid neuroleptization, the most appropriate drug and dose to use is:
   A. Chlorpromazine 200 mg every 4 to 6 hours intramuscularly
   B. Thioridazine 200 mg every 2 hours intramuscularly
   C. Haloperidol 5 to 10 mg intramuscularly every 2 hours until the patient is sedated or less psychotic
   D. Haloperidol 25 mg every 2 hours until the patient is sedated or less psychotic

Case Continued: A regime in which the patient received haloperidol 5.0 mg i.m. every 2 hours until sedated, or was no longer a danger to himself, was begun. Furthermore, the patient was placed under one-to-one nursing surveillance.

Discussion

This case illustrates the technique of rapid neuroleptization. Haloperidol was chosen because it has relatively few anticholinergic or antiadrenergic side effects, and therefore is less dangerous in terms of causing serious hypotension, sedation, cardiac depressant, or cardiac arrhythmic effects when given aggressively. The technique was chosen in this case since this patient appeared in moderate jeopardy of mutilating himself. Certain centers routinely use this technique without specific indications other than the presence of acute psychotic symptoms.

Case Continued: Over the next 6 hours, the patient received three 5-mg injections of haloperidol. By the time of the last injection, he claimed that he was tired and wanted to go to sleep. He also stated that the voices appeared to be fading, but were still present. The patient slept through his first night in the hospital. By morning, he appeared calmer, and although he still felt that his thoughts were being controlled, he stated that he was no longer hearing God tell him to hurt himself.

4. Once a 24-hour dose of haloperidol has been given during rapid intramuscular neuroleptization, the optimal daily oral haloperidol dose should generally be:
   A. Half the 24-hour i.m. dose
   B. Equal to the 24-hour i.m. dose
   C. Twice the 24-hour i.m. dose
   D. Four times the 24-hour i.m. dose

It was decided that the patient would receive haloperidol orally in a dose equal to that which had been given the previous day. Thus, the patient was begun on 5 mg oral haloperidol, t.i.d.

Discussion

The amount of haloperidol given in the first 24 hours of treatment determined the subsequent daily doses of haloperidol given orally. This is a conventional technique used in rapid neuroleptization.

Case Continued: Over the subsequent week, the patient improved considerably on a regimen of haloperidol 15 mg daily, decreasing the need for nursing surveillance and integrating into the milieu of the unit. By the end of 1 week of hospitalization, the patient was more spontaneous and was claiming that God was no longer talking to him. He decided that the force that was controlling his thoughts had found someone else to bother. He still believed that his hallucinations and delusions had been real.

Answers

1. (B)
2. (C)
3. (C)
4. (B)

References

1. Polak, P. and Laycob, L.: Rapid tranquilization. *American Journal of Psychiatry*, 128: 132–135, 1975.
2. Ayd, F. J.: Haloperidol: 15 years of clinical experience. *Diseases of the Nervous System*, 33: 459–469, 1972.
3. Feldman, P. E., *et al.*: Parenteral haloperidol in controlling patient behavior during acute psychotic episode. *Current Therapeutic Research*, 11:362–366, 1969.
4. Man, P. L. and Chen, C. H.: Rapid tranquilization of acutely psychotic patients with intramuscular Haldol and chlorpromazine. *Psychosomatics*, 14: 59–63, 1973.
5. Donlon, P. and Tupin, J.: Overview: Efficacy and safety of rapid neuroleptization. *American Journal of Psychiatry*, 136: 273–278, 1979.
6. Linden, R. and Davis, J.: High- versus low-dose neuroleptics. *Psychiatric Annals*, 12: 769–781, 1982.
7. Rosenblatt, J. E. and Wyatt, R. J.: Are chlorpromazine dose equivalents equivalent in serum? *Journal of Clinical Psychopharmacology*, 1: 91–93, 1981.
8. Tune, L. E., Creese, I., Depaulo, J. R., *et al.*: Clinical state and serum neuroleptic levels measured by radioreceptor assay in schizophrenics. *American Journal of Psychiatry*, 137(2): 187–190, 1980.
9. Casper, R., Garver, D., Dekirmenjian, H., Chang, S., and Davis, J. M.: Phenothiazine levels in plasma and RBC's: Their relationship to clinical improvement in schizophrenia. *Archives of General Psychiatry*, 37: 301–305, 1980.

10. Yesavage, J., Holman, C., Cohn, R., and Lombrozo, L.: Correlation of initial thiothixene serum levels and clinical response. *Archives of General Psychiatry*, 40: 301–304, 1983.

CASE 4: TREATMENT OF A CHRONICALLY RELAPSING SCHIZOPHRENIC PATIENT

John M. is a 28-year-old male chronic schizophrenic patient with a history of accusatory, auditory hallucinations, delusions of control, suspiciousness that he is being followed by the FBI, and the fear that people are whispering about him and calling him a homosexual. The patient has generally been able to function adequately, living a schizoid life alone in a trailer, but recently became extremely anxious for fear of being called a homosexual. He had not been taking any medications for 1 month before his admission. Since perphenazine had been helpful to him previously, it was decided to treat him as an outpatient with oral doses of perphenazine increased to 24 mg per day over a 1-week period.

1. The most likely diagnosis for this patient is:
   A. Paranoid schizophrenic, chronic type
   B. Schizophrenic psychosis
   C. Schizoaffective psychosis
   D. Hysterical psychosis
   E. None of the above
2. The dose of perphenazine used in this case was:
   A. Too high
   B. Acceptable, but probably too high
   C. Too low
   D. Worthy of a malpractice suit

Discussion

Although doses of 25 to 100 mg per day of perphenazine are frequently employed, lower doses, (i.e., 10 to 20 mg per day) are often sufficient to exert an antipsychotic effect.

Case Continued: Over a period of 1 week, the patient's anxiety abated and he became much less preoccupied with imagined aspersions on his masculinity.

3. The improvement in this patient probably represents:
   A. A true drug effect of the perphenazine
   B. A transference cure
   C. A placebo effect
   D. All of the above

Case Continued: A review of the patient's history reveals that he had existed marginally when taking his medication, but was able to be employed. Consistently, when he stopped his medication, a relapse occurred within several weeks to 1 month. Furthermore, his cessation of medication occurred despite his therapist's and family's admonitions against doing so, and was generally motivated by the patient's need to deny his illness.

4. The suggested course of treatment for a patient who repeatedly stops taking his medication and suffers psychotic relapses is:
   A. Fluphenazine hydrochloride orally given each day
   B. Fluphenazine decanoate given intramuscularly every 2 weeks
   C. Fluphenazine enanthate given intramuscularly every 2 weeks
   D. A or B
   E. B or C
5. The most common side effect of fluphenazine enanthate is:
   A. Sedation
   B. Dystonias and parkinsonian symptoms
   C. Hypotension
   D. Agranulocytosis
6. The optimal dose of a long-acting intramuscular antipsychotic agent such as fluphenazine enanthate is:
   A. One quarter of the usual oral clinical dose
   B. Half the usual oral clinical dose
   C. Two times the usual oral dose
   D. Four times the usual oral dose

Case Continued: On the basis of the above information, it was decided to switch the patient to a long-acting and injectable antipsychotic agent, fluphenazine decanoate. An injection of 25 mg was given intramuscularly, with plans for repeated injections every 2 weeks, with the oral haloperidol given in decreasing doses over the next 5 days and then stopped.

Discussion

Since the patient had a long history of discontinuing his medications, it was decided that a trial of a long-acting antipsychotic drug would be attempted as a way of undercutting this tendency. This technique is often used effectively in patients who are on a "drug merry-go-round," and who relapse frequently, since it takes the control of drug-therapeutic compliance out of the patient's hands.

Case Continued: The patient continued to improved. His delusions and hallucinations virtually stopped, and he began to talk of leaving the hospital to return to his home. He began to look for a job and was ultimately rehired by a previous employer. The patient's outpatient physician was urged to continue to give the patient intramuscular fluphenazine decanoate 25 mg every 2 weeks, which he agreed to do. The patient's family were encouraged to report to the treating physician any resurgence of symptoms or tendency to not have an injection as soon as such symptoms occurred. Over the subsequent 6 months the patient has done well, continuing to receive treatment and to work.

Answers

1. (A)
2. (B)
3. (A)
4. (E)
5. (B)
6. (D)

References

1. Beckmann, H.: High dose diazepam in schizophrenia. *Psychopharmacology*, 7: 79–82, 1980.
2. Davis, J. M.: Dose equivalence of the antipsychotic drugs. *Journal of Psychiatric Research*, 2: 65–69.

3. Linden, R. and Davis, J.: High- versus low-dose neuroleptics. *Psychiatric Annals*, 12: 769–781, 1982.
4. Tune, L., Creese, I., Depaulo, J. R., *et al.*: Clinical state and serum neuroleptic levels measured by radioreceptor assay in schizophrenia. *American Journal of Psychiatry*, 137: 187–190, 1980.
5. Brown, W. A., Laughren, T., Chisholm, E., and Williams, B. W.: Low serum level neuroleptic levels predict relapse in schizophrenic patients. *Archives of General Psychiatry*, 39: 998–1000, 1982.
6. Davis, J. M.: Overview: Maintenance therapy in psychiatry: I. Schizophrenia. *American Journal of Psychiatry*, 132: 1237–1245, 1975.
7. Hogarty, G. E. and Ulrich, R. F.: Temporal effects of drug and placebo in delaying relapse in schizophrenic outpatients. *Archives of General Psychiatry*, 34: 297–301, 1977.
8. Gardos, G. and Cole, J. O.: Maintenance antipsychotic therapy: Is the cure worse than the disease? *American Journal of Psychiatry*, 133: 32–36, 1977.

CASE 5: SIDE EFFECTS OF ANTIPSYCHOTIC DRUGS IN A MEDICATION-SENSITIVE PATIENT

A 43-year-old woman with sleeplessness and anxiety and a history of schizophrenia is put on chlorpromazine 400 mg at bedtime. She informs her physician that she is very sensitive to medications and always has bad reactions to "all" medications. True to her statement, she develops maximum side effects from the chlorpromazine.

1. Match the stated mechanism of action with the side effects this patient develops:
   A. Hypotension
   B. A dystonia
   C. Parkinsonian tremor, mask-like face, drooling
   D. Akathisia
   E. Dry mouth
   F. Blurred vision
   G. Constipation
   H. Breast swelling and lactation
   I. A rash
   J. Jaundice
   K. Sleepiness
   L. Seizures

M. A tardive dyskinesia
N. Agranulocytosis
O. A tachycardia
P. Dizziness and fainting
Q. An increased serum prolactin level

(1) Blockade of dopaminergic receptors
(2) Blockade of noradrenergic receptors
(3) Blockade of acetylcholine receptors (anticholinergic effects)
(4) Activation of cholinergic activity
(5) Allergic mechanism
(6) Idiosyncratic
(7) Blockade of dopamine receptors and facilitation of cholinergic activity
(8) Unknown
(9) Dopamine-receptor hyperactivity

2. The danger of seizures developing is decreased if the chlorpromazine is:
   A. Given in a slowly increasing dosage
   B. Given to patients with no preexisting seizure disorder
   C. Given along with an anticonvulsant such as sodium diphenylhydantoin (Dilantin), if a seizure has previously occurred
   D. All of the above
   E. A and C
3. Agranulocytosis frequently presents as:
   A. A sore throat and fever
   B. Muscle aches and pains
   C. Changes in blood color
4. The jaundice caused by chlorpromazine is usually:
   A. Cholestatic
   B. Biliary
   C. Hepatocellular
5. The decreased visual accommodation caused by antipsychotic agents is best treatable by:
   A. Pilocarpine
   B. Store-bought eyeglasses for presbyopia
   C. Eyeglasses for myopia
6. If an allergic rash develops, it is best to:
   A. Begin diphenhydramine (Benadryl) and continue to give the antipsychotic agent

   B. Switch to another antipsychotic drug in the same chemical category
   C. Switch to another antipsychotic drug in another chemical category (substitute a phenothiazine for a thioxanthene, etc.)
7. Chlorpromazine should never be given to:
   A. Patients with a history of liver disease
   B. Patients with cholestatic jaundice
   C. Patients who have a family history of alcoholism
   D. All of the above
   E. None of the above
8. The lethargy and somnolence that can accompany chlorpromazine treatment usually:
   A. Are not severe but are annoying
   B. Disappear with continued antipsychotic drug treatment
   C. All of the above
   D. None of the above
9. Patients who develop a drug-induced dry mouth may respond to:
   A. A cholinergic drug such as bethanechol (Urecholine)
   B. Switching to a less anticholinergic antipsychotic drug, such as haloperidol
   C. Chewing gum
   D. All of the above
   E. None of the above
10. The photosensitivity occurring in patients treated with antipsychotic agents is best prevented by:
   A. Taking vitamin A
   B. Taking vitamin C
   C. Having the patient cover the exposed portion of his body with a sunscreen, long sleeves, a broad-brimmed hat or in some other way

Discussion

The side effects of the antipsychotic medications are quite numerous. Generally, they fall into certain broad etiologic categories. Antinoradrenergic effects probably cause hypotension, dizziness and somnolence. Anticholinergic effects generally cause dry mouth, paralysis of accommodation, and constipation. Dopamine blockade causes an increase in serum prolactin release with associated breast engorgement and lactation. The extrapyramidal effects of antipsychotic medications are due to a blockade of dopamine, associated with an increase in central cholinergic activity. Cholestatic hepatic effects and agranulocytosis appear to be idiosyncratic. Various rashes generally are caused by allergic reactions. Generally, the side effects caused by the antipsychotic agents are treated symptomatically, and by switching to drugs in other chemical subgroups. Thus, for example, parkinsonian side effects may be treated by switching to a more anticholinergic antipsychotic agent such as chlorpromazine, in place of haloperidol or benztropine. Seizures may be treated with anticonvulsant drugs. Photosensitivity can be treated with a sunscreen or protective clothing. Paralysis of accommodation may be treated with eyeglasses. Somnolence may be endured until tolerance develops, or may be antagonized by methylphenidate given in small doses. Similarly, hypotension may respond to a switch to a more potent antipsychotic agent with weaker antinoradrenergic effects, or by administering small doses of sympathomimetic agents, such as methylphenidate or ephedrine. The more serious side effects of antipsychotic drugs, such as agranulocytosis and cholestatic jaundice, are best approached by being alert to their possible occurrence. Both occur very rarely, but their seriousness probably warrants continued vigilance.

Answers

1. (A-2, B-7, C-7, D-8, E-3, F-3, G-3, H-1, I-5, J-6, K-2, L-8, M-9, N-6, O-3, P-2, Q-1)
2. (D)
3. (A)
4. (A)
5. (B)
6. (C)
7. (E)
8. (D)
9. (D)
10. (C)

References

1. Bishop, M. P., Gallant, D. M., and Sykes, T. F.: Extrapyramidal side effects and therapeutic responses. *Archives of General Psychiatry*, 13: 155–162, 1965.

2. Baer, R. L. and Harris, H.: Types of cutaneous reactions to drugs. *American Medical Association*, 202: 710, 1967.
3. Satanove, A.: Pigmentation due to phenothiazines in high and prolonged dosage. *Journal of the American Medical Association*, 191: 262, 1965.
4. Hagopian, V., Stratton, D. B., and Busilla, R. D.: Five cases of pigmentary retinopathy associated with thioridazine administration. *American Journal of Psychiatry*, 121: 1, 1964.
5. DiMascio, A. and Shader, R. I. (eds.): *Clinical Handbook of Psychopharmacology*. Jason Aronson, New York, 1970.
6. Ghadirian, A. M., Chouinard, G., and Annable, L.: Sexual dysfunction and plasma prolactin levels in neuroleptic treated schizophrenic outpatients. *Journal of Nervous Mental Disorders*, 170: 463–467, 1982.
7. Mitchell, J. E. and Popkin, M. K.: Antipsychotic drug therapy and sexual dysfunction in men. *American Journal of Psychiatry*, 139: 633–636, 1982.

CASE 6: MAINTENANCE ANTIPSYCHOTIC DRUG THERAPY

A 24-year-old male is brought in for an evaluation by his family. He recently moved to the city after having experienced, over the last 18 months, two hospitalizations for schizophrenia, paranoid type. The family decided that he might enjoy life better if he lived with his brother, and as a result he has moved to this new location. The patient explains that he is currently taking trifluroperazine (Stelazine) 10 mg, b.i.d. and chlorpromazine (Thorazine) 300 mg, at bedtime. He states that he was last in the hospital approximately 4 months previously, at which time he experienced paranoid delusions and hallucinations. The physical examination is within normal limits. The patient denies auditory hallucinations, delusions, or intrusive thoughts. There is no tangentiality, hallucinations, or looseness of associations. The patient's affect is appropriate and somewhat superficial. There is no disturbance of mood noted, and the patient does not appear depressed. The initial impression is that the patient represents a case of schizophrenia, paranoid type, in remission.

1. The most logical recommendation for treatment at this time would be:
   A. Stop all medications
   B. Decrease all medications by 50%

C. Discourage the patient from his current move and encourage him to return to his former treatment program and home
D. Continue his present medication program and arrange a follow-up visit

2. Research into maintenance antipsychotic drug therapy in schizophrenia has shown:
   A. Continuation of antipsychotic medications is much too dangerous a treatment program to be advocated.
   B. Continuation of medication is statistically unnecessary
   C. Distinct indications exist for who should receive antipsychotic drug maintenance therapy and who should not
   D. Fewer antipsychotic-drug-treated patients, as opposed to placebo-treated patients, experience relapse
3. If a patient with a history of recurring schizophrenic episodes stops taking antipsychotic medications, the chance of relapse in the first year is approximately:
   A. 95%
   B. 65%
   C. 15%
   D. 10%
4. Patients with a history of recurring schizophrenic episodes, receiving antipsychotic medication on a maintenance basis, have the following chance of relapse within 1 year:
   A. 95%
   B. 65%
   C. 45%
   D. 30%
   E. 10%

Discussion

In a review of 24 controlled studies on the use of maintenance antipsychotic drugs, it was observed that for 698 schizophrenic patients out of 1,068 who received placebo, 65% relapsed, in contrast with 639 out of 2,127 (30%) who received maintenance antipsychotic medications. These drugs thus prevented relapse in a substantial number of patients, with the percent relapsing in drug-treated groups being less than that observed in the control group. Maintenance antipsychotic drug treatment is thus indicated for prophylactic purposes in schizophrenic patients with a history of frequent relapse. Generally speaking, the most effective antipsychotic drug for a given patient during the acute phase of his illness is also indicated for maintenance of that patient after remission. Undermedicating a patient during the maintenance phase is as unsound as overmedicating. Clinical and pharmacologic evidence favors a dose range of 200 to 500 mg per day of chlorpromazine or its equivalent for maintenance therapy, although there is a reported wide variation in this figure. Since, in the case described, this is the first clinical encounter, it would seem appropriate that no changes be made in the patient's medication, and that the patient be observed and followed carefully in his new social setting.

5. The diagnostic group least likely to require long-term maintenance therapy with an antipsychotic agent is:
   A. Schizophrenia, chronic undifferentiated type
   B. Schizophrenia, disorganized type
   C. Schizophrenia, paranoid type
   D. Brief, reactive psychosis
   E. Schizophrenia, residual type

Discussion

There is no firm information about whether or not maintenance antipsychotic medications are indicated for patients experiencing a "reactive psychosis." A review of studies of the natural history of reactive psychosis, by such workers as Stevens and Astrup, suggest that the prognosis in these reactive disorders may be fairly good, and that many of these patients do not relapse without medication. Thus, patients with a single schizophrenia-like episode might require, at most, only short-term maintenance treatment to insure a desirable recovery. These patients may represent a group who do well in spite of being on placebos in maintenance therapy studies. This population is quite different from patients with a history of chronic relapsing schizophrenia. The patient discussed in this case had a history of two prior psychotic episodes, which would probably warrant continued drug therapy.

6. Patients with a history of schizophrenia, receiving maintenance antipsychotic medications and with no recurrences within the past 3 years should probably have their medications:

A. Continued
B. Discontinued immediately
C. Tapered
D. Changed to a different medication
E. Increased

Discussion

Now that there is recognition of long-term side effects following antipsychotic drug therapy, it is obviously important to treat patients with the minimal amount of drug necessary for the shortest period, in the hope of preventing tardive dyskinesias. For the patient who has not had a psychotic episode in 3 years, antipsychotic medication should be tapered with the hope of stopping all medication in a 3- to 6-month period. It should be made clear to the patient that the return of any psychotic symptoms, such as hallucinations or delusions, should be brought to the attention of the physician. Patients will frequently experience a great deal of psychologic dependency on a medication program that they have followed for a number of years. However, data suggests that the schizophrenic process may "burn out" in some chronically ill patients. Many chronically ill but remitted patients will ultimately do best when all drugs are withdrawn. Considerations, then, of the patient's chronicity and drug history are relevant in deciding issues regarding inpatient and outpatient maintenance antipsychotic medications.

7. The return of symptoms following discontinuation of maintenance antipsychotic medications usually occurs:
   A. Within 24 hours
   B. Within 3 weeks
   C. Within 2 months
   D. By 6 months and later
   E. At unpredictable intervals

Discussion

Significant numbers of patients relapse when antipsychotic medications are withdrawn. However, this often may not occur until 3 to 6 months or longer after the discontinuation of medication. Therefore, there are no guarantees that discontinuation of medication, and a lack of relapse, can predict a patient's future course. Patients who have had psychotic episodes in the past should be followed for extended periods, even when no antipsychotic medications are being used in their management.

8. Major changes in the patient's current medications may have a significant effect on:
   A. Transference reactions
   B. Counter-transference feelings
   C. The patient's feelings toward the previous doctor
   D. Rescue fantasies
   E. All of the above
9. When starting new medications or changing a medication protocol, telling the patient that he may expect relief, and listing the general areas in which this relief may occur, as well as potential side effects, leads to:
   A. Better results
   B. Poorer results
   C. Increased complaints and enhanced sensitivity to side effects
   D. Apprehension on the part of the patient and resistance to taking the medication
   E. All of the above

Discussion

The patient–therapist–drug relationship is a complicated one. Discontinuing drugs prescribed by other therapists requires careful evaluation, with consideration of the potential effects on prior patient–therapist relationships. It is advisable and pertinent to review in detail the patient's past experience with drugs and to take a careful psychiatric history. There is good experimental evidence that when the physician prescribes an active drug, there will be better results if he potentiates the drug effect by suitably influencing the patient's attitudes and expectations. This may be done, for example, by telling the patient that he may expect relief and listing the general areas in which this relief may occur. Patients should also be carefully informed about the side effects of a given drug, such as drowsiness or dry mouth, and that the side effects may be annoying. Information about the nature, dosage, size, and color of the medication prescribed are also helpful in familiarizing the patient with the medication and having the patient cooperate in his own management.

10. Drug therapy is optimal when:
    A. The patient is in a dependent position
    B. The patient is carefully monitored
    C. The patient feels that he is mutually responsible with the physician for his treatment
    D. The patient feels he is doing what is best for himself

Discussion

Drug therapy should be structured so that the patient himself feels that he is taking responsibility for his existence by making the decision to take the medication. Frequently, participation by the patient in medication decisions is a valuable therapeutic experience in mastery and control, and self-medication is an important part of preparation for discharge from the hospital. When a patient shows no improvement in spite of an expected positive response to a drug program, the possibility that he is not taking his medication must always be considered.

11. Of the following medications, the only agent not available in injectable form is:
    A. Chlorpromazine
    B. Haloperidol
    C. Thioridazine
    D. Imipramine
12. For the average patient, most of the therapeutic gain of receiving an antipsychotic agent occurs in the:
    A. First 2 to 3 weeks
    B. First 4 or 5 weeks
    C. First 6 to 8 weeks
13. In comparing antipsychotic agents, the only drug found to be less effective than chlorpromazine given in equivalent dosages is:
    A. Haloperidol (Haldol)
    B. Thioridazine (Mellaril)
    C. Trifluoperazine (Stelazine)
    D. Promazine (Sparine)
    E. Perphenazine (Trilafon)

14. The significant clinical difference(s) between the phenothiazines, thioxanthines, and butyrophenones is (are):
    A. Onset of action
    B. Site of action
    C. Energizing effect
    D. Side effects
    E. All of the above
15. Match the strengths of the various antipsychotic agents to 100 mg of chlorpromazine:

A. Haloperidol (Haldol)	(1) 100 mg
B. Thiothixene (Navane)	(2) 5.0 mg
C. Thioridazine (Mellaril)	(3) 10 mg
D. Fluphenazine (Prolixin)	(4) 2.5 mg
E. Trifluoperazine (Stelazine)	(5) 2.0 mg

Discussion

The patient who uses activity as a defense mechanism may become quite alarmed upon being sedated. Such a patient usually will do best while receiving nonsedating antipsychotic drugs. Whether or not a given patient responds differentially to a given antipsychotic drug is an empirical question that cannot be adequately answered from existing clinical data. As a matter of clinical course, however, once a drug has been adequately tried for a sufficient period with only minimal to moderate improvement, discontinuing the drug and instituting a drug of a different class, such as a thioxanthene or butyrophenone for a phenothiazine, should be attempted.

Answers

1. (D)
2. (D)
3. (B)
4. (D)
5. (D)
6. (C)
7. (E)
8. (E)
9. (A)
10. (C)
11. (C)
12. (C)
13. (D)
14. (D)
15. (A-5, B-3, C-1, D-4, E-2)

References

1. Davis, J. M.: Overview: Maintenance therapy in psychiatry: I. Schizophrenia. *American Journal of Psychiatry*, 132(12): 1237–1245, 1975.
2. Stephens, J. H. and Astrup, C.: Prognosis and process in non-process schizophrenia. *American Journal of Psychiatry*, 119: 945–953, 1963.
3. Stephens, J. H.: Long-term course and prognosis of schizophrenia. *Seminars in Psychiatry*, 2: 464–485, 1970.
4. Valient, G. E.: Prospective prediction of schizophrenic remission. *Archives of General Psychiatry*, 11: 509–518, 1964.
5. Phillip, R. A.: Schizophrenia: Overview of treatment methods. In: *Comprehensive Textbook of Psychiatry*, Vol. II (eds: A. M. Freedman, H. I. Kaplan, B. J. Sadock). Williams & Wilkins, Baltimore, 1976, p. 935.
6. Rosenblatt, J. E. and Wyatt, R. J.: Are chlorpromazine dose equivalents equivalent in serum? *Journal of Clinical Psychopharmacology*, 1: 91–93, 1981.
7. Smith, R. C., Crayton, J., Dekirmenjan, H., Klass, D., and Davis, J. M.: Blood levels of neuroleptic drugs in nonresponding chronic schizophrenic patients. *Archives of General Psychiatry*, 36: 579–584, 1979.
8. Hogarty, G. E. and Goldberg, S. C.: Drug and sociotherapy in the aftercare of schizophrenic patients. *Archives of General Psychiatry*, 28: 54–64, 1973.
9. Goldberg, S. C., Schooler, N. R., Hogarty, J. E., and Roper, M.: Prediction of relapse in schizophrenic out-patients treated by drugs and sociotherapy. *Archives of General Psychiatry*, 34: 171–184, 1977.

CASE 7: TARDIVE DYSKINESIA IN A CHRONIC SCHIZOPHRENIC PATIENT

A 62-year-old chronic schizophrenic woman who has been a 20-year inpatient in a state mental hospital is noted to manifest bizarre repetitive movements of her mouth, tongue, hands, and feet. Her mouth involuntarily grimaces and her tongue intermittently protrudes. Her fingers repetitively flex and she often is noted to rock back and forth. Her hand and feet movements appear choreiform. The patient has a history of paranoid delusions and hallucinations, beginning 25 years previously. She has not manifested these symptoms of schizophrenia for 6 years. She has been treated with a progression of antipsychotic drugs in moderate doses for the past 18 years. She is currently receiving haloperidol (Haldol) 40 mg per day, benztropine mesylate (Cogentin) 2.0 mg thrice daily, and fluphenazine decanoate (Prolixin) 25 mg i.m. every 2 weeks.

1. The most likely diagnosis for the repetitive movements is:
   A. Tardive dyskinesia
   B. Schizophrenic stereotyped behavior
   C. Conversion reaction
   D. Huntington's chorea
2. The repetitive movements:
   A. Are probably but not always permanent
   B. Are probably temporary
   C. Will probably wax and wane in intensity in parallel with the patient's anxiety level
   D. A and C
   E. B and C
3. The movements usually:
   A. Intensify over time
   B. Bother the patient considerably
   C. Lead eventually to death or paralysis
4. The probable cause(s) of the movements is (are):
   A. Hypersensitivity of dopaminergic neurons in the basal ganglia, caused by chronic dopamine blockade
   B. Chronic antipsychotic drug administration
   C. Genetic
   D. Anticholinergic agents such as benztropine mesylate
   E. A and B
   F. C and D
5. Discontinuation of the patient's antipyschotic medications will probably:
   A. Increase the movements
   B. Decrease the movements
   C. Not change the movements
6. Doubling the dose of haloperidol will:
   A. Decrease the movements
   B. Increase the movements
   C. Cause the underlying neuropathology to increase
   D. A and C
   E. B and C

7. Patients having the following characteristics are most likely to develop tardive dyskinesia:
   A. Intake of antipsychotic drugs for many years
   B. Advanced age
   C. Being female
   D. Having brain damage
   E. All of the above
   F. None of the above
8. The following agents have been said to be useful in alleviating tardive dyskinesias:
   A. Reserpine
   B. Choline
   C. Deanol
   D. Lithium
   E. Haloperidol
   F. Propranolol
   G. Benzodiazepines
   H. All of the above
9. Of those treatments listed in Question 8:
   A. All have been proven effective
   B. None has been proven very effective in all patients
   C. All have been shown to work in most patients
10. The identification of the entity known as tardive dyskinesia led to the suggestion that antipsychotic agents:
    A. Be withdrawn every 4 to 6 months to see if a tardive dyskinesia has developed
    B. Be used very conservatively
    C. Be used in low doses for as short a period as possible
    D. Not be given "promiscuously" for long periods
    E. All of the above
    F. None of the above

Discussion

The patient probably is suffering from a syndrome known as tardive dyskinesia. This syndrome was first described in the early 1960s, but was generally not recognized as a pathologic entity until the late 1960s. The tardive dyskinesias, in extreme cases, consist of repetitive choreiform hand and foot movements, anterior posterior rocking movements, grimacing and smacking of the lips, and intermittent protrusions of the tongue, known as the buccal–facial–lingual syndrome. One or more components of the syndrome may appear. The syndrome resembles Huntington's chorea, and is most common in patients who are female, elderly, have a history of brain damage, and have been treated chronically with antipsychotic agents. The syndrome is the result of chronic antipsychotic drug treatment. It probably, but not certainly, is related to cumulative drug dosage, and can occur with any antipsychotic agent except reserpine. It can occur as soon as 1 to 2 months after the institution of antipsychotic drug treatment, but usually occurs 6 months to 1 or more years after the institution of such treatment. Tardive dyskinesia is currently thought to be due to a basal-ganglionie dopaminergic hypersensitivity phenomenon secondary to chronic dopaminergic blockade by antipsychotic agents. A similar syndrome can occur with L-dopa or amphetamine administration. Increasing dopaminergic blockade by increasing the prescribed antipsychotic agents leads to a temporary cessation of symptoms. However, the underlying neuropathology is increased and eventually the symptoms resume. When antipsychotic agents are withdrawn, the symptoms are unmasked as dopaminergic blockade decreases. Early in the course of development of tardive dyskinesia, signs may disappear if the patient is taken off antipsychotic medications. However, later in the course of the syndrome, the signs of tardive dyskensia become permanent. No effective treatment for tardive dyskinesia has been developed. Resperine, lithium, deanol, choline, propranolol, benzodiazepines, and other drugs are reported effective in some cases, with deanol and choline probably working by increasing cholinergic activity. Antiparkinsonian agents probably increase the signs of tardive dyskinesia by blocking cholinergic tone, but are probably not etiologically involved. The recognition of the phenomenon of tardive dyskinesia has led to a change in psychopharmacologic practice. It is desirable to decrease or discontinue antipsychotic agents after remission from a psychosis, and to reinstate antipsychotic agents when early symptoms of schizophrenia reappear. In those patients given chronic antipsychotic agents so that they may function, a 2- to 4-week "drug holiday" every 4 to 6 months is desirable so that the signs of early onset tardive dyskinesia, which include subtle tongue movements, can be detected.

Answers

1. (A)
2. (D)
3. (A)
4. (E)
5. (A)
6. (D)
7. (E)
8. (H)
9. (B)
10. (E)

References

1. Kazamatsuri, H., Chien, C., and Cole, J.: Therapeutic approaches to tardive dyskinesia. *Archives of General Psychiatry*, 27: 491–499, 1972.
2. Fann, W. E., Davis, J. M., and Janowsky, D. S.: The prevalence of tardive dyskinesia in mental health patients. *Diseases of the Nervous System*, 33: 182–186, 1972.
3. Crane, G. E.: Tardive dyskinesia in patients treated with major neuroleptics. *American Journal of Psychiatry*, 124: 40–48, 1968.
4. Edwards, H.: The significance of brain damage in persistent oral dyskinesia. *British Journal of Psychiatry*, 116: 271–275, 1970.
5. Gardos, G. and Cole, J.: The prognosis of tardive dyskinesia. *Journal of Clinical Psychiatry*, 44: 177–179, 1983.
6. Gualtieri, C. T., Barnhill, J., McGimsey, J., *et al.*: Tardive dyskinesia and other movement disorders in children treated with psychotropic drugs. *Journal of the American Academy of Child Psychiatry*, 19(3): 491–510, 1980.
7. Klawans, H. L., Goetz, C. G., and Perlick, S.: Tardive dyskinesia: Review and update. *American Journal of Psychiatry*, 137: 900, 1980.
8. Crow, T., *et al*: Abnormal involuntary movements in schizophrenia: Are they related to the disease process or its treatment? Are they associated with changes in dopamine receptors? *Journal of Clinical Psychopharmacology*, 2: 336–340, 1982.
9. Jeste, D. and Wyatt, R.: Therapeutic strategies against tardive dyskinesia. *Archives of General Psychiatry*, 38: 803–816, 1982.
10. Casey, D.: Managing tardive dyskinesia. *Journal of Clinical Psychiatry*, 39: 748–753, 1978.
11. Kane, J. and Smith, J.: Tardive dyskinesia: prevalence and risk factors, 1959 to 1979. *Archives of General Psychiatry*, 39: 473–481, 1982.
12. Mukherjee, S., Rosen, A., Cardenas, C., Varia, V., and Olarte, S.: Tardive dyskinesia in psychiatric outpatients. *Archives of General Psychiatry*, 39: 466–469, 1982.

CASE 8: ANTIPSYCHOTIC-DRUG-INDUCED EXTRAPYRAMIDAL SYMPTOMS IN A 28-YEAR-OLD WOMAN

A 28-year-old female schoolteacher develops delusions, hallucinations, ideas of reference, the belief that she can broadcast thoughts, and a flat affect over a 3-week period. She is admitted to an inpatient psychiatric unit and given a daily dose of fluphenazine (Prolixin) of 20 mg at bedtime. Three days after the beginning of the fluphenazine therapy, she appears stiff, exhibits a pill-rolling tremor, drooling, and masklike facies. These symptoms continue, and on the fourth day of therapy she suddenly develops opisthotonos (hyperextension of the neck) and spasms of her left arm. She appears very anxious and says her neck hurts. An injection is given and the physical symptoms remit.

1. The probable cause(s) of the patient's syndrome is (are):
   A. Hysteria
   B. An extrapyramidal reaction
   C. Imagery
   D. The fluphenazine
   E. An extrapyramidal reaction and the fluphenazine
   F. Hysteria and imagery
2. The patient developed:
   A. Pseudoparkinsonism first, a dystonia second
   B. A dystonia first, pseudoparkinsonism second
   C. Akathisia first, a dystonia second
   D. Parkinsonian symptoms only
3. The acute management of the dystonia could include:
   A. Reassurance
   B. Benztropine mesylate (Cogentin) 1.0 mg i.m. or i.v.
   C. Diphenhydramine (Benadryl) 50 mg i.m. or i.v.
   D. All of the above
   E. None of the above
4. The neurochemical mechanism by which the dystonia and the pseudoparkinsonism probably developed involves:
   A. Blockade of dopamine and activation of acetylcholine
   B. Activation of histamine
   C. Blockade of serotonin and activation of norepinephrine
   D. Blockade of norepinephrine

5. The following statement is true:
   A. Dystonias usually develop in the first 2 weeks of antipsychotic drug therapy, and do not usually occur after 1 month of therapy
   B. Pseudoparkinsonism usually lasts from 6 to 8 months
   C. Most patients who develop pseudoparkinsonism also develop dystonias
   D. Dystonias develop as the blood levels of an antipsychotic drug are increasing

Case Continued: After treatment of the acute dystonia with 1.0 mg benztropine mesylate i.m., the patient is begun on 2.0 mg of this drug daily. All extrapyramidal symptoms disappear. The patient complains of mild blurring of her vision and a dry mouth.

6. The anticholinergic side effects of benztropine mesylate suggest its cautious use and preclude its use in a patient with:
   A. Urinary or bladder-neck obstruction
   B. Closed-angle glaucoma
   C. Cardiac arrhythmia
   D. Bowel obstruction
   E. All of the above
   F. None of the above
7. The patient's benztropine mesylate should be continued:
   A. For as long as the patient receives antipsychotic medications
   B. For 6 weeks and then discontinued to see if the extrapyramidal side effects have disappeared
   C. For about 1 week and then discontinued

Case Continued: Five days after treatment has begun, the patient begins to visually hallucinate and pantomime, and loses all sense of orientation.

8. The most likely diagnosis is:
   A. Central anticholinergic syndrome secondary to benztropine mesylate
   B. Schizophreniform disorder
   C. Brain tumor
9. The most rapid treatment for her symptoms is:
   A. Physostigmine (Antilirium)

B. Diazepam (Valium)
C. Chlorpromazine (Thorazine)

Discussion

Extrapyramidal symptoms are a major side effect of antipsychotic drug therapy. Generally, the antipsychotic drugs shift dopaminergic–cholinergic balance toward a cholinergic predominance, causing such extrapyramidal symptoms as pseudoparkinsonism, dystonias, and akathisias. Pseudoparkinsonism consists of a pill-rolling tremor, masklike facies, cogwheeling and rigidity, hypokinesia, and drooling. The symptoms often develop early in treatment and usually disappear after 6 weeks. Dystonias consist of muscle spasms, including pisthotonos, extensor spasms, jaw spasms, and oculogyric crises. These usually occur during the first 2 weeks of antipsychotic drug therapy and decrease after 2 to 3 weeks. They usually occur as antipsychotic drug blood levels are falling. Akathisias consist of an internal restlessness, associated with anxiety and pacing. All the above extrapyramidal effects are treatable with antiparkinsonian drugs including trihexyphenidyl (Artane), benztropine mesylate, procyclidine (Kemadrin), or amatadine (Symmetrel). The dystonias are often painful and frightening. They are best treated with 1 to 2 mg benztropine mesylate i.m. or 50 mg diphenhydramine (Benadryl) i.v. or i.m. The pseudoparkinsonism symptoms are more benign and are treated by 1 to 6 mg of antiparkinsonian agent each day, except for amatadine (Symmetrel), which is administered in a dose of 100 mg two or three times a day. Similar treatment is indicated for the akathisias. For the above extrapyramidal symptoms, most psychopharmacologists agree that the antiparkinsonian agents should be withheld until symptoms develop, since not all patients develop extrapyramidal symptoms. Some authors, however, believe that for antipsychotic drugs with a high incidence of extrapyramidal side effects, an antiparkinsonian agent should be used initially. Since tolerance to the parkinsonian side effects of antipsychotic agents usually develops by 6 weeks after starting antipsychotic drug therapy, it is wise to discontinue antiparkinsonian agents at 6 weeks and reinstitute them only if the extrapyramidal symptoms recur. Antiparkinsonian agents have strong anticholinergic properties. They are thus contraindicated in patients with bowel or bladder-neck obstruction and closed-angle glaucoma. They can cause an organic brain syndrome with confusion, visual, and auditory hallucinations and agitation, especially in elderly patients. This central anticholinergic syndrome is treatable with i.m. physostigmine (Antilirium).

Answers

1. (E)
2. (A)
3. (D)
4. (A)
5. (A)
6. (E)
7. (B)
8. (A)
9. (A)

References

1. Orlov, P., Kasparian, G., DiMascio, A., and Cole, J. O.: Withdrawal of antiparkinsonian drugs. *Archives of General Psychiatry*, 25: 410–412, 1971.
2. Anjus, J. W. S. and Simpson, G. M.: Hysteria and drug-induced dystonia. *Acta Psychiatrica Scandinavica*, 212: 52–58, 1970.
3. DiMascio, A.: Toward a more rational use of antiparkinsonian drugs in psychiatry. *Drug Therapy*, 1: 23–29, 1971.
4. Sheppard, C. and Merlis, S.: Drug-induced extrapyramidal symptoms: Their incidence and treatment. *American Journal of Psychiatry*, 123: 886–889, 1967.
5. Baldessarini, R. J. and Tarsy, D.: Dopamine and pathophysiology of dyskinesis induced by antipsychotic drugs. In *Annual Review of Neuroscience*, Vol. 3 (ed.: W. M. Cowan). Annual Reviews, Inc., Palo Alto, CA, 1980, p. 23.

CASE 9: THE NEED FOR ANTIPSYCHOTIC DRUG MAINTENANCE IN A YOUNG WOMAN WITH TARDIVE DYSKINESIA

Judith R. is a 27-year-old white unmarried Jewish woman who presented with a history since age 18 of having intermittent psychotic episodes. Although premorbidly a rather shy person, she was able to finish high school. However, during her first college year, she felt she could not cope, felt homesick, and was extremely anxious. In addition, she began to experience vague paranoid symptoms and ideas of reference. As a result, she subsequently dropped out of school and returned home. The next 10 years were spent with attempts to re-enter college or to work at clerical jobs. She had intermittent psychotic episodes, mostly punctuated by paranoid ideation about people casting aspersions on her. In May 1983, the patient and her parents moved to another state, where she continued to live with them. She was frequently disturbed by hearing voices calling her name in a derogatory way. She associated hearing the voices with being stupid, ugly, and incompetent, as well as with previous sexual activities she had engaged in and which she considered immoral. An initial mental-status examination revealed a well-nourished, attractive, alert, well-dressed woman appearing younger than her age. She appeared moderately anxious, and said she was very scared by hearing voices. She showed constriction of affect, was shy, spoke without elaboration, and said she was somewhat depressed. She stated that she was mildly suicidal and displayed autistic thinking. She also displayed mild to moderate mouth, tongue, and hand movements indicative of a tardive dyskinesia. A diagnosis of paranoid schizophrenia, chronic type, was made.

1. In this patient's case, given the existence of her tardive dyskinesia, further use of a dopamine-blocking antipsychotic drug, such as chlorpromazine, haloperidol, or fluphenazine is:
   A. Absolutely contraindicated, based on recent ethical and legal decisions
   B. Dependent of the risk–benefit ratio
   C. Absolutely indicated as a means of preventing psychologic deterioration
   D. In the domain of the psychiatrist to decide
2. This patient's symptoms of tardive dyskinesia are:
   A. Definitely irreversible
   B. Almost certainly irreversible
   C. Possibly irreversible
   D. Very transient

Case Continued: In spite of the patient's tardive dyskinesia, she, her parents, and her psychiatrist elected to begin antipsychotic drug therapy since her psychotic and anxious symptoms were disabling and extremely painful to her, and were severe enough to make the need for hospitalization likely if they continued. The patient was informed of the danger that the antipsychotic drugs would eventually be likely to increase her symptoms of tardive dyskinesia. However, even though such drugs are needed to help the patient stay out of the hospital and to relieve ego-dystonic disabling psychotic symptoms, such drugs might ultimately increase or make more permanent her tardive dyskinesia symptoms. Since, if noticed early, such symptoms can often be reversed by stopping antipsychotic drug treatment, and later can become "fixed," the continued use of these drugs has important implications. However, the risk of having tardive dyskinesia or making it worse must be weighed against the risk of psychosis. The patient and her family were included in the decision-making, and the implications of the dilemma were outlined in detail.

Case Continued: Trifluoperazine (Stelazine) was begun in a 5-mg dosage, t.i.d., and gradually increased over a 1-month period to 15 mg, t.i.d. The gradual dosage increase was implemented because at lower doses the patient's symptoms were only partially alleviated. Early in the course of treatment, the patient developed parkinsonian symptoms, manifested primarily as akinesia and rigidity.

3. In patients with symptoms of tardive dyskinesia who are given an antiparkinsonian agent such as benztropine mesylate or trihexyphenidyl, the symptoms usually:
   A. Intensify
   B. Decrease
   C. Stay the same
4. In patients with symptoms of tardive dyskinesia who are given an antiparkinsonian agent, the underlying lesion responsible for the dyskinesia is:
   A. Made worse
   B. Unchanged
   C. Improved

Discussion

Benztropine mesylate was employed in this patient to treat parkinsonian symptoms caused by the anticholinergic blocking properties of trifluoperazine. Although an anticholinergic drug such as benztropine mesylate can cause an apparent increase in the symptoms of tardive dyskinesia due to a shifting of dopamine-acetylcholine balance in a dopaminergic direction, no fundamental harm to the tardive dyskinetic process apparently occurs when an anticholinergic–antiparkinsonian agent is administered.

5. Risk factors associated with the development of tardive dyskinesia include:
   A. Advancing age
   B. Female sex
   C. Chronic use of any one of the dopamine-blocking antipsychotic drugs
   D. All of the above
   E. A and B
6. Which of the following drugs is least likely to cause tardive dyskinesia:
   A. Chlorpromazine
   B. Haloperidol
   C. Thioridazine
   D. Fluphenazine
   E. Trifluoperazine
   F. None of the above
7. Drug holidays are useful in:
   A. Preventing tardive dyskinesia
   B. Unmasking tardive dyskinesia
   C. Treating tardive dyskinesia
   D. None of the above

Discussion

Overall, prevalence surveys of tardive dyskinesia have found a rate of 20% in antipsychotic-drug-treated individuals. Risk factors associated with this increasingly important public health issue include advancing age and, to a lesser degree, female sex. Interestingly, increasing length of neuroleptic exposure, type of drug, or dose of drug, is not obviously linked with the risk of tardive dyskinesia. Animal studies, however, suggest that certain antipsychotic drugs may be less likely than others to cause tardive dyskinesia. However, such claims are based on very limited animal studies, and probably bear little if any relationship to the development of tardive dyskinesia in humans. No clinical studies have shown any significant differences between drug class in terms of risk of causing tardive dyskinesia; all marketed antipsychotic drugs except reserpine have been reported to be associated with the development of this side effect. Initially it was thought that drug-free intervals would be advantageous in terms of decreasing total drug exposure and consequent development of tardive dyskinesia. Comparative studies, however, have not shown that this practice is advantageous except to unmask tardive dyskinesia.

Answers

1. (B)
2. (C)
3. (A)
4. (B)
5. (D)
6. (F)
7. (B)

References

1. Jeste, D. and Wyatt, R.: Changing epidemiology of tardive dyskinesia: An overview. *American Journal of Psychiatry*, 138: 297–309, 1981.
2. Gardos, G. and Cole, J.: The prognosis of tardive dyskinesia. *Journal of Clinical Psychiatry*, 44: 177–197, 1983.
3. Klawans, H., Goetz, C., and Perlick, S.: Tardive dyskinesia: Review and update. *American Journal of Psychiatry*, 137: 900–908, 1980.
4. Itil, T. M. and Soldatos, C.: Epileptogenic side effects of psychotropic drugs. *Journal of the American Medical Association*, 244: 1460–1463, 1980.
5. Synder, S. H., Greenberg, D., and Yamamura, H. I.: Antischizophrenic drugs and brain cholinergic receptors: Affinity muscarinic sites predicts extrapyramidal effects. *Archives of General Psychiatry*, 31: 58–61, 1974.
6. Kaskey, G. B., Nasr, S., and Meltzer, H. Y.: Drug treatment in delusional depression. *Psychiatry Research*, 1: 267–277, 1980.
7. Charney, D. S. and Nelson, J. C.: Delusional and nondelusional unipolar depression: Further evidence for distinct subtypes. *American Journal of Psychiatry*, 138: 328–333, 1981.
8. Mandel, M., Severe, J., Schooler, N., Gelenberg, A., and Mieske, M.: Development and prediction of post-psychotic depression in neuroleptic-treated schizophrenics. *Archives of General Psychiatry*, 39: 197–203, 1982.

9. Van Putten, T. and May, P.: "Akinetic depression" in schizophrenia. *Archives of General Psychiatry*, 35: 1101–1107, 1978.
10. Baldessarini, R. J. and Tarsy, D.: Dopamine and the pathophysiology of dyskinesis induced by antipsychotic drugs. In: *Annual Review of Neuroscience*, Vol. 3 (ed.: W. M. Cowan). Annual Reviews, Inc., Palo Alto, CA, 1980, p. 23.
11. Beckmann, H.: High-dose diazepam in schizophrenia. *Psychopharmacology*, 7: 79–82, 1980.
12. Jimenson, D., van Kammen, D. P., Post, R. M., Docherty, J. P., and Bunney, W. E., Jr.: Diazepam in schizophrenia: A preliminary double-blind trial. *American Journal of Psychiatry*, 139(4): 489–491, 1982.

CASE 10: NEUROLEPTIC-WITHDRAWAL-INDUCED PSYCHOTIC AND MOVEMENT DISORDERS IN A SCHIZOPHRENIC PATIENT

A 39-year-old white male patient has developed mild hand movements and buccal–facial–lingual movements, indicative of tardive dyskinesia. The patient has a history of having been receiving trifluoperazine (Stelazine) 30 mg per day for 1 year for treatment of his fourth psychotic episode, diagnosed as undifferentiated schizophrenia. He has been almost asymptomatic for 3 months, having only vague suspiciousness as a target symptom.

1. If the patient's medications are decreased to zero over a 2-week period, his tardive dyskinesia symptoms at that time will probably:
   A. Increase
   B. Decrease
   C. Stay the same
2. If the patient's medications are rapidly decreased and he quickly becomes psychotic again, the cause(s) of the psychosis is (are) likely to be:
   A. An unmasking of the underlying psychosis, which has been suppressed by the antipsychotic medications
   B. A "tardive psychosis" that is transient, due to the unmasking of up-regulated dopamine receptors
   C. A and B
   D. None of the above

Discussion

When a patient's chronically administered antipsychotic drugs are rapidly withdrawn, symptoms of tardive dyskinesia often increase, probably due to withdrawal "rebounding" caused by the unmasking of up-regulated dopamine receptors. A parallel phenomenon, also probably due to the unmasking of up-regulated dopamine receptors, is called tardive psychosis, and may represent a withdrawal phenomenon rather than an unmasking of underlying and suppressed psychotic symptoms. A very slow decrease in the antipsychotic drug dose is suggested, so as to avoid "withdrawal psychosis." This psychosis is a psychologic parallel to tardive dyskinesia. Here an antipsychotic drug presumably causes the up-regulation of dopamine receptors in brain areas relevant to the psychosis, and these receptors are unmasked upon abrupt drug withdrawal, leading to a dopamine-induced activation of the psychosis.

3. Treatments that have shown at least some promise in alleviating the symptoms of tardive dyskinesia include:
   A. The use of drugs that activate γ-aminobutyric acid (GABA) activity, such as sodium valproate
   B. The use of lithium
   C. The use of benzodiazepines
   D. The use of clonidine
   E. Choline or lecithin administration
   F. None of the above
   G. All of the above

Discussion

Because tardive dyskinesia often persists after drug discontinuation, or because drugs must be continued, the clinician should be familiar with some of the strategies attempted in the treatment of this dyskinesia. Continuation of treatment with the antipsychotic agent(s) responsible for this syndrome is not generally recommended because of increased long-term risk. Drugs that activate GABA activity, as a group, appear somewhat effective in decreasing the symptoms of tardive dyskinesia. Results with cholinergic drugs such as choline and lecithin have been less impressive than originally hoped for, although the development of more specific preparations may result in increased rates of improvement. Other drugs, such as diazepam, clonidine, and propranolol have also been shown to be of benefit in some patients with tardive dyskinesia. Anticholinergic drugs are of little if any benefit in the treatment of such dyskinesia, and may increase the symptoms. At present, there is no consistently effective treatment for tardive dyskinesia.

Answers

1. (A)
2. (C)
3. (G)

References

1. Chouinard, B. and Jones, B.: Neuroleptic-induced supersensitivity psychosis: Clinical and pharmacologic characteristics. *American Journal of Psychiatry*, 137: 16–21, 1980.
2. Weinberger, D. R., Bieglow, L. B., Klein, S. T., and Wyatt, R. J.: Drug withdrawal in chronic schizophrenic patients: In search of neuroleptic-induced supersensitivity psychosis. *Journal of Clinical Psychopharmacology*, 4: 120–123, 1981.
3. Simpson, G., Varga, E., and Haher, E. J.: Psychotic exacerbations produced by neuroleptics. *Diseases of the Nervous System*, 37: 367–369, 1976.
4. Gardos, G. and Cole, J.: The prognosis of tardive dyskinesia. *Journal of Clinical Psychiatry*, 44: 177–179, 1983.
5. Klawans, H., Goetz, C., and Perlick, S.: Tardive dyskinesia: Review and update. *American Journal of Psychiatry*, 137: 900–908, 1980.
6. Smith, J. M.: Abuse of antiparkinsonian drugs: A review of the literature. *Journal of Clinical Psychiatry*, 41: 351–354, 1980.
7. Schrodt, G. R., Wright, J. H., Simpson, R., Moore, D. P., and Chase, S.: Treatment of tardive dyskinesia with propranolol. *Journal of Clinical Psychiatry*, 43(8): 328–331, 1982.
8. Jeste, D. and Wyatt, R.: Therapeutic strategies against tardive dyskinesia. *Archives of General Psychiatry*, 38: 803–806, 1982.
9. Casey, D.: Managing tardive dyskinesia. *Journal of Clinical Psychiatry*, 39: 748–753, 1978.
10. Kane, J. and Smith, J.: Tardive dyskinesia: Prevalence and risk factors, 1959 to 1979. *Archives of General Psychiatry*, 39: 473–481, 1982.

11. Mukherjee, S., Rosen, A., Cardenas, C., Varia, V., and Olarte, S.: Tardive dyskinesia in psychiatric outpatients. *Archives of General Psychiatry*, 39: 466–469, 1982.

CASE 11: INDICATIONS FOR SPECIFIC ANTIPSYCHOTIC DRUGS IN AN ELDERLY PATIENT

An elderly 74-year-old white woman with a history of hypertension, myocardial infarctions, and ischemic cerebrovascular disease is admitted to the inpatient unit of a university teaching hospital. The woman has a 40-year-long history of recurrent delusions, hallucinations, and ideas of reference. She currently is hallucinating and delusional. She is diagnosed as having paranoid schizophrenia. Her first-year psychiatric resident wishes to begin her on oral thioridazine (Mellaril), planning to gradually increase the dose to 400 mg per day. The faculty member—chief of the unit—suggests that the patient receive oral haloperidol (Haldol), gradually increasing the dose to 10 mg per day. Before drug treatment can be instituted, the patient signs out against medical advice.

1. The best antipsychotic agent for this patient would be:
   A. Reserpine
   B. Thioridazine (Mellaril)
   C. Chlorpromazine (Thorazine)
   D. Haloperidol (Haldol)
2. The reason haloperidol is most efficacious is because it:
   A. Requires the lowest dose
   B. Has the least hypotensive effects
   C. Is less likely to cause extrapyramidal effects
   D. Causes more sedation
3. The greatest danger in using thioridiazine in the above patient would have been:
   A. Its soporific effects
   B. Its hypotensive effects
   C. Its constipating effects
   D. Its tendency to cause ventricular arrhythmias
   E. Its ability to cause retinitis pigmentosa

4. In a young, healthy, agitated, sleepless schizophrenic patient, thioridazine might have been indicated due to its:
   A. Soporific effects
   B. Relative lack of parkinsonian side effects
   C. Neither of the above
   D. Both of the above
5. When an antipsychotic agent with hypotensive, soporific, and anticholinergic properties is used, it is advantageous to:
   A. Begin treatment at the estimated efficacious dose
   B. Gradually increase the dose over a 3- to 7-day period to the estimated efficacious dose
   C. Never exceed the dose recommended in the *Physicians' Desk Reference*
6. If thioridazine were chosen, the highest acceptable dose would be:
   A. 200 mg per day
   B. 400 mg per day
   C. 800 mg per day
   D. 1,600 mg per day
7. The drug most likely to cause seizures in patients with or without a history of seizures is:
   A. Trilafon (perphenazine)
   B. Mellaril (thioridazine)
   C. Thorazine (chlorpromazine)
   D. Haldol (haloperidol)
8. The probability of seizures occurring during antipsychotic drug treatment increases with:
   A. High daily dosages
   B. Rapid increases in dosage
   C. A history of seizures
   D. Withdrawal from a barbiturate treatment
   E. All of the above
   F. None of the above
9. Match the lettered generic names with the numbered brand names:

A. Chlorpromazine	(1) Sparine
B. Trifluoperazine	(2) Mellaril
C. Thioridazine	(3) Stelazine
D. Perphenazine	(4) Trilafon
E. Fluphenazine	(5) Repoise

F. Butaperazine (6) Prolixin
G. Promazine (7) Thorazine

Discussion

In general, the various antipsychotic drugs all are equally efficacious in the treatment of schizophrenic symptoms; no consistent data have indicated that any one agent is more useful in the treatment of a given subgroup of schizophrenia than another, given equivalent dosages. Thus, 500 mg of thioridazine is generally as efficacious as 10 mg haloperidol. The major indication for using a specific antipsychotic agent is the agent's side effects. Basically, two clusters of side effects exist: haloperidol, fluphenazine, trifluoperazine, and butaperazine have predominantly extrapyramidial side effects. Chlorpromazine and thioridazine have a predominant side-effect complex consisting of hypotension, sedation, and anticholinergic symptoms. Overlap between these two clusters exists. Thiothixene and perphenazine have both sets of side effects, although these may be weaker for either cluster. Elderly patients who have cerebrovascular or cardiovascular disease are generally best treated with haloperidol or related agents, so that hypotensive episodes may be avoided. Patients who would be frightened or hindered by extrapyramidal symptoms are best treated with a more soporific drug, such as chlorpromazine. In general, antipsychotic drugs should be slowly increased in dosage until they are effective. However, certain side effects may limit this procedure. For example, thioridazine, given in doses above 800 mg per day, may cause retinitis pigmentosa. Too rapid an increase in chlorpromazine to too high a dose will increase the likelihood of seizures. Too rapid an increase or too high a dose of thioridazine may lead to ventricular arrhythmias. Slowly increasing the dose of an antipsychotic agent decreases the above risks and leads to the identification of side effects while they are mild.

Answers

1. (D)
2. (B)
3. (B)
6. (C)
7. (C)
8. (E)

4. (D)
5. (B)
9. (A-7, B-3, C-2, D-4, E-6, F-5, G-1)

References

1. Hollister, L. E., Overall, E., Kimbell, I., Jr., and Pokorny, A.: Specific indications for different classes of phenothiazines. *Archives of General Psychiatry*, 30: 94–99, 1974.
2. Galbrecht, C. R. and Klett, C. J.: Predicting response to phenothiazines: The right drug for the right patient. *Journal of Nervous and Mental Disorders*, 147: 173–183, 1968.
3. Snyder, S. H., Banerjee, S. P., Yamamura, H. I., and Greenberg, D.: Drugs, neurotransmitters and schizophrenia. *Science*, 184: 1243–1253, 1974.
4. Fitzgerald, C. H.: A double blind comparison of haloperidol with perphenazine in acute psychiatric episodes. *Current Therapeutic Research*, 11: 515–519, 1969.
5. Hogarty, G. E. and Goldberg, S. C.: Drug and sociotherapy in the aftercare of schizophrenic patients. *Archives of General Psychiatry*, 28: 54–64, 1973.
6. Hollister, L. E. and Kim, D. Y.: Intensive treatment with haloperidol of treatment-resistant chronic schizophrenic patients. *American Journal of Psychiatry*, 139: 1466–1473, 1982.
7. Snyder, S. H.: Dopamine receptors, neuroleptics and schizophrenia. *American Journal of Psychiatry*, 138(4): 460–464, 1981.
8. Itil, T. M. and Soldatos, C.: Epileptogenic side effects of psychotropic drugs. *Journal of the American Medical Association*, 244: 1460–1463, 1980.
9. Hollister, L. E.: Antipsychotic medications and the treatment of schizophrenia In: *Psychopharmacology: From Theory to Practice* (eds.: J. D. Barchas, P. A. Berger, R. D. Ciaranello, and G. R. Elliott). Oxford University Press, New York, 1977, p. 121.

CASE 12: DEVELOPMENT OF TARDIVE DYSKINESIA IN AN ELDERLY PATIENT

A 65-year-old chronic schizophrenic woman who has been hospitalized for 20 years is discharged from a state hospital. She comes to treatment at the local community mental health center complaining that her tongue keeps sticking out, her jaw moves involuntarily, and that her fingers tend to open and close. Her sensorium and orientation are clear and she is not hallucinating or delusional.

1. The most likely cause of this patient's movements is:
   A. Huntington's chorea
   B. Schizophrenic stereotyped movements
   C. Tardive dyskinesia
   D. Hemiballismus

Case Continued: The patient announces that for the past 10 years she has received high doses of various tranquilizers to control the "demons" and voices she hears, and has recently had her medications stopped. A call to the state hospital reveals that she has sequentially received numerous phenothiazines and butyrophenones.

2. It is most likely that the patient's movements will:
   A. Increase with a reduction of the antipsychotic drug dosage
   B. Remit if the antipsychotic drug dose is increased
   C. Ultimately get worse if the dose is increased
   D. A and C
   E. All of the above
   F. None of the above
3. If antipsychotic drugs are stopped completely, it is likely that this patient's dyskinetic movements will eventually:
   A. Diminish
   B. Disappear
   C. Stay the same after an initial increase
4. The most effective treatment listed below for alleviation of the symptoms of tardive dyskinesia, without ultimately aggravating the symptoms, is probably:
   A. Haloperidol
   B. Reserpine
   C. Guanethidine
   D. Phenobarbital
5. The identification of the entity known as tardive dyskinesia led to the suggestion that antipsychotic agents:
   A. Be withdrawn every 4 to 6 months to see if a tardive dyskinesia has developed

B. Be used very conservatively
C. Be used in low doses for as short a period as possible
D. Not be given indiscriminately for long periods
E. All of the above
F. None of the above

Discussion

Tardive dyskinesia is a disfiguring, often irreversible side effect of long-term antipsychotic drug use. It consists of dyskinetic movements of the mouth, tongue, extremities, fingers, and back, and can be disabling. Buccal–facial–lingual movements and hand and finger movements are regular manifestations. The symptoms tend to occur in elderly females, but can occur in males and in younger individuals. Symptoms can occur after a few months of antipsychotic drug therapy, but usually occur after at least 6 months to 1 year of treatment. The effects are not frequently irreversible, although symptoms can be suppressed by increasing the antipsychotic drug dosage. This, however, ultimately increases the symptoms. Antipsychotic drug withdrawal increases the symptoms. There is no standard effective treatment, although lithium carbonate, reserpine, benzodiazepines, propranolol, and deanol have been reported useful. The identification of the tardive dyskinesias has caused a rethinking of the use of antipsychotic agents, leading to their more conservative usage.

6. The basis for the development of tardive dyskinesia is thought to be:
   A. Dopamine-receptor hypersensitivity
   B. Dopamine-receptor hyposensitivity
   C. Norepinephrine-receptor hypersensitivity
   D. Acetylcholine-receptor hyposensitivity

Discussion

Based on previous findings, the likely basis of tardive dyskinesia is dopamine hypersensitivity. This hypersensitivity is caused by a receptor up-regulation following chronic receptor suppression, which in effect causes a "denervation hypersensitivity."

7. If dopaminergic hypersensitivity is the cause of tardive dyskinesias, chemical models of therapeutic intervention could be:
   A. Drugs that deplete dopamine at the synapse
   B. Drugs that cause dopamine blockade
   C. Both
   D. Neither

Discussion

Dopamine-depleting drugs such as reserpine, tetrabenazine, and alpha-methyldopa all deplete available catecholamines, and therefore have been tried with marginal effectiveness in tardive dyskinesia. Dopamine-blocking drugs such as the antipsychotics (phenothiazines and butyrophenones) have been shown to have antidyskinetic efficacy. Unfortunately, they also further intensify the underlying tardive dyskinesia. Other psychotropic agents, such as monoamine oxidase inhibitors, have also been tried.

8. Antiparkinsonian agents such as trihexyphenidyl (Artane) and benztropine mesylate (Cogentin):
   A. Are effective in treating tardive dyskinesia
   B. Have no effect in tardive dyskinesia
   C. May aggravate the symptoms of tardive dyskinesia

Discussion

Anticholinergic agents, such as trihexyphenidyl and benztropine mesylate have been known to potentiate the effect of dopamine at the synapse. They may also intensify the probable neurochemical imbalance occurring in tardive dyskinesia by blocking cholinergic receptors.

Answers

1. (C)	5. (E)
2. (E)	6. (A)

3. (C)
4. (B)
7. (C)
8. (C)

References

1. Kazamatsuri, H., Chien, C., and Cole, J. O.: Therapeutic approaches to tardive dyskinesia. *Archives of General Psychiatry*, 27: 491, 1972.
2. Christensen, E., Møller, J. E., and Faurbye, A.: Neuropathological investigation of 28 brains from patients with dyskinesia. *Acta Psychiatrica Scandinavica*, 46: 14–23, 1970.
3. Baldessarini, R. J. and Tarsy, D.: Dopamine and the pathophysiology of dyskinesis induced by antipsychotic drugs. In: *Annual Review of Neuroscience*, Vol. 3 (ed.: W. M. Cowan). Annual Reviews, Inc., Palo Alto, CA, 1980, p. 23.
4. Crow, T., *et al.*: Abnormal involuntary movements in schizophrenics: Are they related to the disease process or its treatment? Are they associated with changes in dopamine receptors? *Journal of Clinical Psychopharmacology*, 2: 335–340, 1982.
5. Schrodt, G. R., Wright, J. H., Simpson, R., Moore, D. P., and Chase, S.: Treatment of tardive dyskinesia with propranolol. *Journal of Clinical Psychiatry*, 43: 328–331, 1982.
6. Jeste, D. and Wyatt, R.: Changing epidemiology of tardive dyskinesia: An overview. *American Journal of Psychiatry*, 138: 297–309. 1981.
7. Gardos, G. and Cole, J.: The prognosis of tardive dyskinesia. *Journal of Clinical Psychiatry*, 44: 177–197, 1983.
8. Klawans, H., Goetz, C., and Perlick, S.: Tardive dyskinesia: Review and update. *American Journal of Psychiatry*, 137: 900–908, 1980.

CASE 13: USE OF RESERPINE IN A CHRONIC SCHIZOPHRENIC PATIENT

A 58-year-old female patient has a history of gradually progressive psychologic deterioration over the past 25 years, and symptoms consistent with a chronic schizophrenic disorder. She has no history of significant depressive disease. She has been intermittently maintained on various antipsychotic drugs for 10 years and has definitely improved while receiving these medications. She currently has no hallucinations and only occasionally has mild delusions and symptoms of a thought disorder. She comes to her community psychiatric outpatient clinic wishing to stop her currently administered haloperidol (Haldol) 10 mg, q.i.d. because she has read about and fears that she will develop tardive dyskinesia if she continues taking the drug.

1. If the patient stops her medication, it is likely she will:
   A. Remain in good psychologic control
   B. Improve
   C. Relapse
2. A rational alternative to completely stopping her medication is to:
   A. Switch her to another antipsychotic medication and tell her it is safe
   B. Discontinue her medication completely every other year
   C. Send her to a hypnotist
   D. None of the above
3. A rational alternative to completely stopping her medication is to:
   A. Switch to reserpine
   B. Switch to propranolol
   C. Switch to chlordiazepoxide (Librium)
   D. Begin alpha-methyldopa (Aldomet)
4. If the patient accepts the choice of being switched to reserpine, this is a rational choice because:
   A. Reserpine is a relatively good antipsychotic agent that probably does not cause tardive dyskinesia
   B. Reserpine doesn't cause too many side effects
   C. Reserpine is a derivative of a plant root, and thus is morally better than a chemical
5. The side effects of reserpine include:
   A. Hypotension
   B. Nausea and vomiting
   C. Diarrhea
   D. Depression
   E. Impotence
   F. Lethargy

G. All of the above
H. None of the above

6. The side effects of reserpine are caused by:
   A. Increased cholinergic and decreased noradrenergic central activity
   B. Increased cholinergic and decreased noradrenergic peripheral activity
   C. Increased cholinergic and decreased noradrenergic central and peripheral activity
   D. Decreased noradrenergic activity alone
   E. Decreased cholinergic activity alone
7. The side effects of reserpine:
   A. Are generally overestimated
   B. Are generally underestimated
   C. Seem in reasonable perspective
   D. Are not important
8. Depression usually occurs with reserpine administration:
   A. In 5 to 15% of treated cases
   B. During chronic reserpine administration, weeks to months after beginning a course of treatment
   C. Most often in patients who have a history of significant depressive disease
   D. None of the above
   E. All of the above

Discussion

In patients with a history of chronic schizophrenia who have been asymptomatic for many years, a trial period without antipsychotic medications may be indicated, since at least one study indicates that many such patients will not relapse upon drug withdrawal. However, in chronically schizophrenic patients with controlled but observable symptoms, continued maintenance antipsychotic drug therapy is indicated. The possibility of tardive dyskinesia presents a dilemma in the treatment of such patients. Decreasing the dose of medications to the minimum that will control symptoms is a reasonable course of action in such cases.

However, a less popular but rational treatment of such chronic patients is to switch them to reserpine. Although reserpine generally is not used in American psychiatry, this drug represents a useful antipsychotic agent which, however, is somewhat less effective than chlorpromazine. Reserpine has not been shown to cause tardive dyskinesia, and may in fact decrease such symptoms. Its use is associated with numerous side effects, including hypotension, nausea, vomiting, diarrhea, lethargy, impotence, and depression. Such effects are generally due to a decrease in noradrenergic activity and an increase in cholinergic activity centrally and peripherally. The side effects of reserpine, especially depression, are generally overrated. The side effects of other antipsychotic agents are more often ignored or minimized by physicians. Generally, reserpine-induced depression, if it should occur, occurs in patients with a preexisting history of depression. It occurs late in a course of therapy. In a general population of patients, it will occur in 5 to 15% of cases. It can be significant, leading at the extreme to serious depression, treatable with antidepressant drugs or electroconvulsive therapy (ECT). Thus, reserpine represents a reasonable alternative to the use of the phenothiazines and related antipsychotic compounds. Its use is associated with significant side effects, which should be carefully monitored. These side effects do not preclude its use.

Answers

1. (C)
2. (D)
3. (A)
4. (A)
5. (G)
6. (C)
7. (A)
8. (E)

References

1. Lewy, A. J. and Goodwin, F. K.: Mental effects of reserpine in man. In: *Psychiatric Complications of Medical Drugs* (ed.: R. I. Shader). Raven Press, New York, 1979.
2. Nasrallah, H. A., Risch, S. C., and Fowler, R. C.: Reserpine, serotonin, and schizophrenia. *American Journal of Psychiatry*, 136: 856–857, 1979.

CASE 14: TAPERING OF ANTIPSYCHOTIC DRUGS IN A RELAPSE-SENSITIVE PATIENT

A 48-year-old woman has a history of schizophrenia, paranoid type, with autism, delusions, and hallucinations. She was last treated at a hospital with haloperidol (Haldol) 40 mg per day. Her discharge prescription from the hospital was for one 10-mg haloperidol tablet per day, which she has taken regularly for 6 months. Her previous psychiatric history has shown that she frequently relapses into psychosis within 1 week of stopping her medication.

1. With regard to this patient's management, which of the following statements is true?
   A. This patient's medication should not be changed
   B. A slow decrease in medication is indicated, with close monitoring for recurrence of psychiatric symptoms
   C. A "drug holiday" should be started, in which this patient's medications are stopped for 1 month
   D. An anticholinergic agent should be added to the regime
2. The dilemma posed by this patient is that:
   A. She needs her antipsychotic medication to function, yet risks developing tardive dyskinesia
   B. She has a choice of behaving like a "zombie" on drugs or becoming psychotic again off drugs
   C. She will have to sacrifice her sleep habits to attain an antipsychotic effect

Discussion

A current dilemma in psychopharmacology involves the chronic use of antipsychotic agents in patients who have been shown to relapse when these agents are withdrawn. The dilemma lies in the fact that long-term antipsychotic drug administration may prevent psychotic decompensation, but can lead to tardive dyskinesia. Since patients often can be maintained on lower doses of antipsychotic agents than are needed to treat an acute psychosis, it is probably worthwhile to slowly taper a patient's antipsychotic medication intake over a period of months. This may decrease the risk of tardive dyskinesia. Certain patients may respond well to remarkably low doses of antipsychotic agents (e.g., 25 mg chlorpromazine per day), and yet rapidly relapse when the drug is withdrawn completely.

Answers

1. (B)
2. (A)

References

1. Rifkin, A., *et al.*: Long-term use of antipsychotic drugs. In: *Progress in Drug Treatment*, Vol. I (eds.: D. F. Klein and R. Gittelman-Klein). Brunner/Mazel, New York, 1975, pp. 387–396.
2. Chien, C. P. and DiMascio, A.: Clinical effects of various schedules of medication. *Behavioral Neuropsychiatry*, 3: 5–9, 1971.
3. Leff, J. P. and Wing, J. K.: Trial of maintenance therapy in schizophrenia. *British Medical Journal*, 3: 599–604, 1971.
4. Mandel, M., Severe, J., Schooler, N., Gelenberg, A., and Mieske, M.: Development and prediction of post-psychotic depression in neuroleptic-treated schizophrenics. *Archives of General Psychiatry*, 39: 197–203, 1982.
5. Van Putten, T. and May, P.: "Akinetic depression" in schizophrenia. *Archives of General Psychiatry*, 35: 1101–1107, 1978.
6. Chouinard, G. and Jones, B.: Neuroleptic-induced supersensitivity psychosis: Clinical and pharmacologic characteristics. *American Journal of Psychiatry*, 137: 16–21, 1980.
7. Weinberger, D. R., Bieglow, L. B., Klein, S. T., and Wyatt, R. J.: Drug withdrawal in chronic schizophrenic patients: In search of neuroleptic-induced supersensitivity psychosis. *Journal of Clinical Psychopharmacology*, 4: 120–123, 1981.
8. Simpson, G., Varga, E., and Haher, E. J.: Psychotic exacerbations produced by neuroleptics. *Diseases of the Nervous System*, 37: 367–369, 1976.
9. Kessler, K. A. and Waletzky, J. P.: Clinical use of the antipsychotics. *American Journal of Psychiatry*, 138: 202–209, 1981.

SECTION II
AFFECTIVE DISORDERS

CASE 15: TREATMENT OF UNIPOLAR DEPRESSION

A 48-year-old woman presents with a 2-month history of sadness, initial and terminal insomnia, lethargy, inability to do her work or concentrate, and a lack of interest in her activities. The symptoms began in the midst of some marital difficulties, but persisted despite an improved home situation. The patient is a sad-appearing, soft-spoken woman without makeup but neatly dressed. She was brought in by her husband, who became concerned when she began talking about suicide. She has no past history of psychiatric disorders.

1. In light of this history, the possible diagnoses include:
   A. Bipolar disorder
   B. Schizophrenia, disorganized type
   C. Alcoholism
   D. Generalized anxiety disorder
   E. Major depression

Discussion

While it is not possible to be certain of the diagnosis, there are guidelines that help to rule in or rule out the diagnoses mentioned above. Schizophrenia of the disorganized type has a slow onset, usually lacks affective symptoms, and has, as its central symptomatology, problems of thinking. Generalized anxiety disorder is a symptom complex centering around anxiety attacks (usually described as taking the form of palpitations, shortness of breath, overwhelming anxiety, and complications of hyperventilation, beginning usually in the teens or 20s, and almost always by age 30). Thus, neither of these diagnoses would be tenable in this patient. Affective disorder and alcoholism are both possibilities here, as each can present with a primary picture of affective changes occurring with a fairly clear onset.

2. You decide that the diagnosis is major depressive disorder. The treatments that have been proven to be effective in decreasing symptoms of this disorder include:
   A. Chlorpromazine (Thorazine)
   B. Amitriptyline (Elavil)
   C. Chlordiazepoxide (Librium)
   D. Electroconvulsive therapy

Discussion

While many therapies have been recommended for the affective disorders, there are few that have appeared effective in controlled studies. There is no indication that the major tranquilizers such as chlorpromazine, or the minor tranquilizers such as chlordiazepoxide (with the possible exception of alprazolam) are useful in treating the core symptoms of affective disorder. These agents may, however, lower anxiety level of the affectively ill patient. The treatments of choice for unipolar depression include the tricyclic antidepressants, such as amitriptyline (Elavil) and imipramine (Tofranil), the newer antidepressants, and electroconvulsive therapy (ECT). The monoamine oxidase inhibitors (MAOIs) are also effective in treating this syndrome.

3. You choose to administer imipramine (Tofranil). Temporary side effects the patient is likely to experience include:
   A. Blurred vision
   B. Diarrhea
   C. Lethargy
   D. Amenorrhea

Discussion

No central-nervous-system (CNS)-altering drug should be given without adequate indications for its use, since they all have significant side effects. At the same time, however, once a decision is made that the institution of these drugs is warranted, they should be given in large enough doses to be effective. If too-small doses are used, one is only exposing the patient to the side effects of the drug without allowing a good chance for recovery. The most frequently encountered side effects of the tricyclic antidepressants are relatively benign. They include the anticholinergic symptoms of dry mouth (in 20 to 40% of patients), constipation (10 to 30% of patients), urinary retention (5 to 10% of patients), and disturbed vision-especially blurring (10 to 20% of patients). In addition, lethargy is frequently reported.

4. General guidelines for the administration of imipramine include:
   A. It is most effective if given in divided daily doses
   B. The average patient will require 150 mg or more daily for a clinical response to occur
   C. Side effects correlate very closely with blood levels
   D. Older patients may require lower doses than younger ones

Discussion

The tricyclic antidepressants have a relatively long half-life, and accumulate in the body. The average patient will require 150 to 300 mg daily for a clinical response to occur. It is the practice of a number of investigators to give a single daily dose about 1 hour prior to sleep. Most patients tolerate this well, and the number of side effects experienced during the day are usually considerably lessened, while there is no indication that such dosage decreases the effectiveness of the treatment. No close correlation between side effects and drug blood levels has been demonstrated, although the number of pharmacokinetic investigations done has been quite limited, and weak trends exist.

5. Correct statements about the tricyclic antidepressants include:
   A. Imipramine is an energizing drug
   B. Amitriptyline is the best tricyclic for the treatment of menopausal depressions
   C. Amitriptyline is contraindicated in a patient with documented heart disease
   D. If the patient responded to a given drug in a past depression, she is likely to respond to the same drug again

Discussion

There are a number of generalizations about the tricyclic antidepressants which are useful to keep in mind. While some of the drugs (such as imipramine) have less sedative properties than others (such as amitriptyline), these drugs are generally not energizing agents, as are the psychostimulants. In addition, all of the tricyclic antidepressants are basically equivalent in efficacy, and none has been shown to be superior to the others for the treatment of any subtype of affective disorder in controlled studies. While these drugs have side effects, and must be used carefully in subsets of patients, such as those with heart disease, they are not contraindicated for such patients. Another general rule is that, if a patient has responded to a drug in the past, that drug should probably be used for subsequent depressions, since it probably has the highest chance of effectiveness.

Answers

1. (A and E)
2. (B and D)
3. (A and C)
4. (B and D)
5. (D)

References

1. Jackson, J. E. and Bressler, R.: Prescribing tricyclic antidepressants. Part I. General considerations. *Drug Therapy*, 11: 87, 1981.
2. Bielski, R. J. and Friedel, R. O.: Prediction of tricyclic antidepressant response: A critical review. *Archives of General Psychiatry*, 33: 1479–1489, 1976.
3. Richelson, E.: Pharmacology of antidepressants in use in the United States. *Journal of Clinical Psychiatry*, 43, (11, Section 2): 4–11, 1982.
4. Berger, P.: Antidepressant medications and the treatment of depression, In: *Psychopharmacology: From Theory to Practice* (eds.: J. Barchas, P. Berger, R. Ciaranello, and G. Elliott). Oxford University Press, New York, 1977, pp. 174–207.
5. Schildkraut, J. J., *et al.*: The catecholamine hypothesis of affective disorders: A review of supporting evidence. *American Journal of Psychiatry*, 122: 509–522, 1965.

6. Schildkraut, J. J., *et al.*: Laboratory tests for discrimination of subtypes of depressive disorders based on measurements of catecholamine metabolism. In: *Affective and Schizophrenic Disorders: New Approaches to Diagnosis and Treatment* (ed.: R. Zales). Brunner/Mazel, New York, 1983, pp. 103–123.
7. Ayd, F.: New antidepressant drugs. *Psychiatric Annals*, 11: 11–17, 1981.
8. Hollister, L.: Plasma concentrations of tricyclic antidepressants in clinical practice. *Journal of Clinical Psychiatry*, 43(2): 66–69, 1982.

CASE 16: TREATMENT OF A CASE OF DEPRESSION WITH IMIPRAMINE

Mrs. O. is a 35-year-old white mother of two with a 10-year history of chronic feelings of dissatisfaction, irritability toward her children and husband, and periods of withdrawal and lethargy, associated with sadness and crying. Although these symptoms have generally worsened during the 3 to 5 days prior to her menstrual periods, they have occurred intermittently and generally lasted from several days to several weeks. The patient's family history is significant in that her father and sister had a history of unipolar, recurrent depression. During the year prior to evaluation, Mrs. O. began a trial of psychotherapy with a licensed family therapist, who saw her weekly and treated her with a reality-oriented psychotherapeutic approach. The patient had told a marriage-and-family counselor that 1 year earlier the patient's father, who was a physician, had given her imipramine in doses of 150 mg per day, and that these had made her feel less irritable and energic after a period of 8 days. However, she had discontinued the imipramine after 3 weeks because she did not want to take medication, nor did she want her father to be in any way in control of her life. The patient said that she felt she was ready for another such trial of an antidepressant "on her own terms."

1. The drug choice for this patient is imipramine because:
   A. It is relatively nonsedating
   B. It has previously proven useful in this patient
   C. It has proven useful in a first-degree relative of the patient
   D. A and C
   E. B and C

2. The need for an antidepressant in this patient probably is:
   A. Nil
   B. Indicated
   C. Equivocal
   D. None of the above

Discussion

Imipramine (Tofranil) is indicated in this patient because this drug had been used successfully by her father, and specific drug effectiveness often appears genetically linked. In addition, the patient had used imipramine in the past, with positive results.

Case Continued: One week later, the patient was begun on a trial of imipramine 50 mg daily, with the dose increased to 50 mg twice daily after 3 days. One week after starting the imipramine, the patient returned for evaluation. She reported having a moderately dry mouth and constipation. Her dose of imipramine was increased over the next week to 50 mg orally, t.i.d. On a subsequent return visit the patient said she had felt less irritable and more relaxed for about 3 days. The imipramine was increased to 200 mg orally at bedtime. One week later the patient returned, saying she felt much better and attributing her improvement to the imipramine. She stated that she was no longer lethargic or irritable, and was less prone to feel picked on by her husband. She still complained of constipation and having a dry mouth.

3. The optimal dose of imipramine in an average-sized young woman is usually:
   A. 50 to 100 mg per day
   B. 100 to 150 mg per day
   C. 150 to 200 mg per day
   D. 200 to 250 mg per day

Discussion

A frequent mistake, made especially by nonpsychiatric physicians, involves giving too low a dose of antidepressant. Often, a dose of 200 to 250 mg per day or more is required for such antidepressants as imipramine or amitriptyline. Such doses are often higher than those suggested in the *Physicians' Desk Reference.*

4. If a patient develops peripheral anticholinergic side effects with a tricyclic antidepressant, the options for treatment include:
   A. Lowering the drug dose
   B. Administering urecholine
   C. Waiting for tolerance to develop
   D. All of the above

Case Continued: A trial of urecholine 10 mg, q.i.d. was begun with alleviation of the anticholinergic target symptoms. At this point it was agreed that the patient would see the psychopharmacologist every 4 weeks, and would be monitored between these visits by her psychotherapist.

Discussion

Since the patient developed bothersome anticholinergic effects, trial therapy with bethanechol (urecholine), a peripherally acting cholinomimetic drug that antagonizes peripheral anticholinergic effects, such as dry mouth and constipation, was instituted. Alternatively, a decrease in drug dosage or the eventual development of tolerance may alleviate such symptoms.

Case Continued: Two months later, feeling much less irritable and not depressed, the patient expressed a wish to try a less potently anticholinergic drug. Her imipramine was tapered over a 1-week period and a trial of desipramine was simultaneously begun, with doses increased over 1 week to 200 mg p.o. at bedtime. However, after 1 week of this treatment the patient had insomnia, felt jittery, and was depressed once again. For this reason the imipramine was restarted and increased to 200 mg per day, and the desipramine was stopped. The patient improved again over the next week and elected to not re-start her urecholine treatment.

5. When an antidepressant is withdrawn and symptoms of anxiety, depression, agitation, insomnia, nightmares, and gastrointestinal hyperactivity develop over several days, this most often is due to:

A. Recurrence of the depression
B. Unmasking of up-regulated acetylcholine receptors, leading to "cholinergic overdrive"
C. Unmasking of the underlying depression

Answers

1. (E)
2. (C)
3. (D)
4. (D)
5. (B)

References

1. Rounsaville, B. J., Klerman, G. L., and Weissman, M. M.: Do psychotherapy and pharmacotherapy for depression conflict? *Archives of General Psychiatry*, 38: 24–55, 1981.
2. Bialos, D., *et al.*: Recurrence of depression after discontinuation of long term amitriptyline treatment. *American Journal of Psychiatry*, 139: 325, 1982.
3. Gillin, J. C., Duncan, W., Pettigrew, K. D., Frankel, B. L., and Snyder, F.: Successful separation of depressed and insomniac subjects by EEG sleep data. *Archives of General Psychiatry*, 36: 85–90, 1979.
4. Veith, R. C.: Urinary MHPG excretion and treatment with desipramine or amitriptyline: Prediction of response, effect of treatment and methological hazards. *Journal of Clinical Psychopharmacology*, 3: 18–27, 1983.
5. Paykel, E. S., Rowan, P. R., Parker, R. R., and Bhat, A. V.: Response to phenelzine and amitriptyline in subtypes of outpatient depression. *Archives of General Psychiatry*, 39: 1041–1049, 1982.
6. Janowsky, D. S., Curtis, G., Zisook, S., *et al.*: Ventricular arrhythmias possibly aggravated by trazodone. *American Journal of Psychiatry*, 140: 796–797, 1983.
7. Rickels, K. and Case, J.: Trazodone in depressed outpatients. *American Journal of Psychiatry*, 139: 803–806, 1982.
8. DiMascio, A., Weissman, M. M., Prusoff, B. A., *et al.*: Differential symptom reduction by drug and psychotherapy in acute depression. *Archives of General Psychiatry*, 36: 1450, 1979.
9. Rush, J. A., Beck, A. T., Kovacs, M., Weissenburger, M. A., and Hollon, S. D.: Comparison of the effects of cognitive therapy and pharmacotherapy on hopelessness and self-concept. *American Journal of Psychiatry*, 139: 862, 1982.

10. Rickels, K., Csanalosi, I., Werblowsky, J., *et al.*: Amitriptyline–perphenazine and doxepin in depressed outpatients: A controlled double-blind study. *Journal of Clinical Psychiatry*, 43:419–422, 1982.

CASE 17: DIFFERENTIATION OF DEMENTIA VERSUS PSEUDO-DEMENTIA

An appointment is made with your office by a patient calling with complaints of "memory problems" and "lack of energy". Mr. S. arrives at your office for his appointment. He appears well dressed but very perplexed and worried. He gives a history that at 80 years of age he is the last remaining member of his family. He states that approximately 7 months ago, the last of his siblings, a sister, passed away in the Midwest. It was 2 years ago that Mr. S. himself was widowed. He gives a history of increasing difficulty in caring for himself. He states that his memory is not the way it used to be and he is upset that he cannot think as clearly as he had previously. In addition to your interview with Mr. S., you also interview his son at the patient's request. The son states that his father had actually functioned quite well until about 6 months ago. He goes on to explain that he had been active in various pursuits, and in fact had continued to work effectively on a part-time basis. He then began losing interest and began complaining that he "wasn't the man I used to be." He said that his relationship with his girlfriend had deteriorated at that time, and he began losing confidence and interest in routine responsibilities, such as driving his car and going to the office where he worked as an accountant. He complained that he could not keep track of the figures, and that he was worried that he would make a mistake. Mr. S. complains a great deal about his physical state, describing a variety of aches and pains and morbid concerns about dying. A history reveals that there has been no previous experience of a psychiatric disorder, such as depression, and that there is no record in the patient's family of dementia. A mental-status examination is characterized by a continued need for reassurance. The patient often tells the examiner that he simply can't cooperate in the examination because he "can't think straight," saying "My memory isn't what it used to be." After continued support and questioning, however, answers that the patient could not provide seem to be found. When asked where he was born, he responds, "It was a small town. I'm not even sure I can remember the name," but then goes on to give both the town name and the address of his childhood home. When asked his current address and telephone number, he states, "I can't worry about things like that." His fund of knowledge seems adequate but is difficult to access since the patient frequently answers with superficial or abbreviated responses. When asked about certain current events, he expands on them, but only with reassurance. Further clinical information shows that the patient seems to improve as the day goes on, with the mornings being "impossible." He states that he has little energy and does not want to get out of bed, finding it difficult to organize his thoughts for the day. You inquire about his recent medical examination and the patient says that he was fully examined only 30 days ago and that his internist felt he was quite healthy. He is currently receiving no medications.

1. The most important feature of the mental status examination is:
   A. The patient's continued complaint of cognitive dysfunction
   B. That the patient answers questions correctly with reassurance and persistance
   C. The presence of ruminations and obsessions
   D. The presence of paranoid thinking

Discussion

The differentiation of dementia from pseudo-dementia caused by depression is an important diagnostic issue in geropsychiatry. Patients with pseudo-dementia complain of cognitive loss, and provide such complaints in detail. They emphasize their disability, highlight their failures, and make little effort to perform tasks, communicating a strong sense of distress. Their actual behavior may be incongruent with the severity of their cognitive dysfunction, and improves as the day goes on. Dementia is contrasted by few complaints of cognitive loss and an attempt to disguise any deficit with jargon, social superficialities, or even hostility and defensiveness. The patient's complaints of cognitive dysfunction are usually vague in dementia, and there is an attempt to conceal the disability. At times the demented patient may even highlight his or her accomplishments, no matter how minimal, and struggle to perform tasks. Affect is frequently labile and shallow rather than dramatic and depressed. Characteristically, the symptoms appear to worsen as the day goes on, owing to the patient's fatigue contributing to the reduced cognitive capacity.

Case Continued: The patient's onset of symptoms appears to have occurred over the previous 6 months. There is also a clear-cut history of the patient being functional until a series of stresses related to the loss of his sister and other losses contributed to his present difficulties.

Discussion

In pseudo-dementia the family is frequently aware of the dysfunction and its severity, whereas in dementia the process is insidious, with the family unaware. In pseudo-dementia the onset can be dated with some degree of accuracy, and a history of previous psychiatric dysfunction may be common. In dementia, previous psychiatric difficulties are unusual.

Case Continued: The family states that before seeing you they had been told by the internist that there was a high possibility that Mr. S. was experiencing the onset of senile dementia of an Alzheimer's type.

2. Pseudo-dementia is infrequently confused with true dementia:
   A. True
   B. False

Discussion

Pseudo-dementia is believed to be present in at least 10% of the geriatric population thought to have dementia. It is reversible with appropriate treatment. Pseudo-dementia may also be superimposed upon true dementia. A diagnosis of dementia in an individual who in fact, has serious cognitive difficulties may lead to that person's disposition to a custodial-care facility, while the diagnosis of pseudo-dementia due to depression might lead to treatment and maintenance of the individual at a higher level of functioning. Most geriatric patients have impaired concentration, memory, and orientation when depressed. They frequently manifest a disorder of motivation and energy, and defensive answers such as, "I don't know," or "I don't remember," making the examiner particularly aware of the amotivational features of depression.

Case Continued: A further history reveals that Mr. S. has had a poor appetite and significant weight loss over the previous 3 months. There have also been episodes of both insomnia and hypersomnia, agitation, decreased libido, and increasing feelings of worthlessness and guilt. At this point treatment with an antidepressant medication is recommended.

3. Which of the following statements is least correct concerning antidepressant medication:
   A. Psychotherapy in conjunction with medication is an appropriate treatment
   B. Antidepressants are of little benefit in the presence of "pure" senile dementia
   C. Cardiovascular side effects such as hypotension in an 80-year-old patient are a serious concern
   D. Antidepressants can be used at the same dosage in a patient of this age as in younger patients

Discussion

Some authors feel that as many as 30% of individuals with primary dementia have a serious affective disturbance. Antidepressants have proven to be quite effective in such cases. The starting dose of the drug should be about one third of the usual dose.

4. Which of the following antidepressants has the fewest active metabolites?
   A. Nortriptyline
   B. Amitriptyline
   C. Imipramine

Discussion

Nortriptyline, desipramine, and protriptyline do not have active metabolites. Protriptyline can at times cause heightened agitation in the elderly. Nortriptyline and desipramine seem to be quite effective and appear to cause fewer side effects.

Case Continued: You choose an antidepressant medication, and approximately 4 days after the initiation of therapy you are called by the family stating that Mr. S. is becoming increasingly confused and disorganized. He has begun to visually hallucinate and is describing events that have not occurred, according to his son, with whom he is temporarily residing.

5. The most probable cause of these events is:
   A. Escalation of the patient's depression to include delusional features
   B. Toxicity caused by the medication
   C. Precipitation of a dementing process under strain
   D. Alcohol abuse

Discussion

With the presence of visual hallucinations and a rapid deterioration in the patient's functional level shortly after the initiation of antidepressant medication, the most common cause would be a central anticholinergic syndrome. Furthermore, recent studies have shown that a tricyclic-antidepressant-induced central anticholinergic syndrome with delirium, resulting from the antimuscarinic properties of these agents, may not be significantly more frequent in the elderly than in the general population. Signs of anticholinergic toxicity, such as temperature elevation, tachycardia, nocturnal confusion, visual hallucinations, and fluctuations in memory and orientation must be monitored. In the event that these reactions occur, discontinuation of the antidepressant usually leads to recovery in 24 to 48 hours and the discontinuation of Mr. S.'s medication at this time would be appropriate. The presence of visual hallucinations suggests toxicity. A further evaluation for possible toxins, such as learning about Mr. S.'s use of alcohol would be pertinent and important. However, and again, it would be an unlikely source of the deterioration in this particular case.

6. Which one of the following tests would be most helpful at this time?
   A. Thyroid level
   B. Dexamethasone suppression test
   C. Serum level of antidepressant
   D. CBC

Discussion

Blood-level measurements of antidepressant medications have considerably improved the treatment of depression. Studies have shown that in patients over 60 years old who develop a toxic syndrome, a blood level of 400 ± 75 ng/ml is not uncommon. Where possible, blood-level readings for these drugs should be obtained 7 to 10 days after the initiation of antidepressant therapy, especially in older patients. It is not uncommon, for instance, that a medication such as nortriptyline will produce an initial improvement and then accumulate to toxic levels. It is also not uncommon for older patients to initially do well on medication and subsequently, as a consequence of medical difficulties, such as dehydration or cardiac problems, to begin to accumulate a drug that they had previously maintained at a lower steady-state level in their plasma.

Case Continued: Mr. S., after a 72-hour period, has shown progressive improvement in his mental functioning. However, he remains depressed, and you are asked to help.

7. Your next therapeutic decision should be:
   A. To recommend electroconvulsive therapy
   B. To reinstitute an antidepressant
   C. To use stimulants

Discussion

An antidepressant medication, at a lower dosage and with less anticholinergic potency, is recommended. If you had previously used doxepin or amitriptyline, which have relatively stronger anticholinergic properties, a drug such as trazodone, desipramine, or nortriptyline might have a lesser potential for toxicity. Electroconvulsive therapy has been shown to be safer than the use of tricyclic antidepressants or monoamine oxidase inhibitors. The patient might be comfortably managed on a lower-dosage antidepressant medication program. In some individuals the direct use of stimulants has been helpful. However, stimulant medications may lead to anxiety or to a rebound depression at a later time.

Answers

1. (B)
2. (B)
3. (D)
4. (A)
5. (B)
6. (C)
7. (B)

References

1. Janowsky, D. S.: Pseudo-dementia in the elderly: Differential, diagnosis and treatment. *Journal of Clinical Psychiatry*, 43(9, Section 2): 19–25, 1982.
2. Wells, C. E.: Pseudo-dementia. *American Journal of Psychiatry*, 136(7): 895–900, 1979.
3. Meyers, D. S. and Mei-Tal, V.: Psychiatric reactions during tricyclic treatment of the elderly reconsidered. *Journal of Clinical Psychopharmacology*, E(1): 2–6, 1983.

CASE 18: TREATMENT OF A CASE OF RESISTANT DEPRESSION

Mrs. H. is a 38-year-old married white woman with two school-age children, and is a registered nurse. Her formal psychiatric history began at age 28, at which time she began a series of hospitalizations for depression and suicidal ideation, receiving diagnoses of recurrent depression, borderline personality, and schizoaffective disorder. During her initial weekly sessions, Mrs. H. gave a history of having been depressed virtually all of her life. She spoke of extreme parental disapproval and criticism, of withdrawing into a fantasy world as a child, and of having felt and feeling worthless, hopeless, and useless, as well as chronically sad since at least early adolescence. Furthermore, Mrs. H. felt that she was being judged by others, and that she had to be perfect in all her activities to prevent being criticised. She spoke of being obsessive about plans and details in her life, and at times was incapacitated by her ruminations over small details. During her mental-status examination, Mrs. H. appeared to be a tired, drab, and untidily dressed woman wearing no make-up, and was sad and cried easily. She expressed feelings of hopelessness, worthlessness, and uselessness, and was preoccupied with "doing a good job." She expressed some suicidal ideation, but said that she would not commit suicide owing to her strong Catholic religious commitment, although she wished she could do so. She spoke of dying as a release from the bonds of her life and illness.

1. The most likely diagnosis (diagnoses) for this patient is (are):
   A. Major depressive disorder
   B. Dysthymic disorder
   C. Both of the above
   D. None of the above

Discussion

Recent information suggests that a patient may have a lifelong history of depression in the form of a dysthymia or "neurotic depression," and at the same time have a formal diagnosis of major depressive disorder. Such a syndrome may be treatable with antidepressant drugs.

Case Continued: Over the next several weeks the patient showed moderate improvement. She ceased to be desirous of dying, and showed some humor, yet she still felt quite depressed. There ensued a discussion, spanning several sessions, of whether or not to try antidepressant medication, with the patient fearing the use of drugs and feeling she should be able to get herself together without such "crutches." Finally, it was mutually agreed that the patient would begin a trial course of treatment with an antidepressant. Ultimately, a trial of amoxapine was begun. The patient received one 50-mg dose without ill effects. By 1 week after starting amoxapine, she was receiving a dose of 50 mg, q.i.d. without side effects other than a dry mouth.

2. Amoxapine is relatively unique as an antidepressant in that it has:
   A. Anticonvulsant properties
   B. Dopamine-blocking properties
   C. Stimulant properties
   D. None of the above
3. Amoxapine can cause:
   A. Akathisias

B. Parkinsonian symptoms
C. Tardive dyskinesia
D. Dystonias
E. All of the above
F. None of the above

Discussion

Amoxapine has dopamine-blocking properties, and as such is unique among the tricyclic antidepressants in causing extrapyramidal symptoms. Such symptoms can include dystonias, akathisias, Parkinsonian symptoms, and in rare instances, tardive dyskinesia.

Case Continued: By the sixth day of treatment, the patient noted that she was feeling somewhat better, less sad, less obsessive, more optimistic, and more outgoing. By the second week of therapy she said that she felt the best she had ever felt in her life, and that her whole outlook had changed. She stated that things that had bothered her before no longer did so, and that she was feeling hopeful. She dressed in more colorful clothes for her psychiatric appointment, seemed bright-eyed, was only mildly depressed, and was no longer suicidal. She displayed a good sense of humor. She attributed these changes to the medication.

4. In a patient such as this, the characterologic features and chronicity of symptoms indicate that:
   A. Interpersonal therapies are solely indicated
   B. Antidepressant drug therapy is solely indicated
   C. A and B are indicated
   D. Electroconvulsive therapy is indicated

Discussion

The many characterologic qualities in this case could have led a therapist to believe that interpersonal therapy rather than somatic therapy was solely indicated. However, the patient did not respond maximally to interpersonal therapy, and did have symptoms of a major depressive disorder. An open-minded approach to this patient allowed for use of antidepressant drugs along with a psychotherapeutic approach.

Case Continued: At the next weekly session, the patient parenthetically asked if the medication could cause a rash. She then displayed a maculopopular rash which covered most of her body. She reported that her face had been swollen and that the rash had progressed over a 3-day period. The patient had not reported the rash for fear that the medication would be stopped. She also reported nausea, diarrhea, and vague joint pains. A visit to a dermatologist led to the diagnosis of a drug-allergy reaction, with possible serum sickness, and the medication was discontinued. Considering the seriousness of the patient's symptoms, a further trial of amoxapine was obviously not warranted.

5. If a patient develops an allergic reaction to a tricyclic antidepressant, it is best to:
   A. Stop all drugs and switch to psychotherapy
   B. Switch to a chemically unrelated compound such as a monoamine oxidase inhibitor or trazodone
   C. Switch to a different tricyclic antidepressant

Case Continued: Over a 4-week period without medication, the patient's depressive symptoms gradually recurred until she was as she had been prior to starting drug therapy. She was unhappy about the recurrence of her symptoms, but her optimism continued since she was told that if one drug had worked, another probably would also be helpful. Ultimately, a trial of monoamine oxidase inhibitor (MAOI) was decided upon, since these drugs are chemically unrelated to amoxapine. The side effects of MAOIs, including the potential for hypertensive crises, were discussed with the patient. The possibility of developing hypotension and sedation was also stressed. After several weeks of discussion, and after the patient had decided that the risks were worth the potential benefits, a trial of phenelzine (Nardil) was begun.

6. The most common serious side effect of an MAOI such as phenelzine is:
   A. Hypertension
   B. Hypotension
   C. Sleepiness
   D. Nausea
   E. Insomnia
7. MAOIs have been shown useful in treating:
   A. Panic attacks

B. Atypical depression
C. Depression in the elderly
D. Bipolar depression
E. All of the above

Discussion

Despite being notorious for causing hypertensive crises, the MAOIs most commonly cause hypotension. Other side effects of these drugs include sedation, insomnia, agitation, nausea, vomiting, and diarrhea. In addition, some evidence has suggested that MAOIs may be especially indicated in geriatric depression, panic attacks, atypical depression, and bipolar depression.

Case Continued: A list of restricted foods and medications was given to the patient. The patient was started on phenelzine 15 mg per day. Since no serious side effects occurred, the phenelzine dose was increased to 15 mg, t.i.d. over a 2-week period. After 10 days of therapy the patient's symptoms had begun again to remit. A further decrease in depressive symptoms occurred over a 2- to 3-week period.

Discussion

A trial of amoxapine was effective in this patient, approximately within the expected time course of action for symptom alleviation beginning 1 to 2 weeks after starting therapy. The development of a serious allergic reaction precluded further use of this drug. A switch to phenelzine, which is not chemically related to amoxapine, was chosen to avoid further allergic reactions.

Answers

1. (C)
2. (B)
3. (E)
4. (C)
5. (B)
6. (B)
7. (E)

References

1. Richelson, E.: Pharmacology of antidepressants in use in the United States. *Journal of Clinical Psychiatry*, 43: 4–11, 1982.
2. Veith, R. C.: Urinary MHPG excretion and treatment with desipramine or amitriptyline: Prediction of response, effect of treatment and methological hazards. *Journal of Clinical Psychopharmacology*, 3: 18–27, 1983.
3. Paykel, E. S., *et al.*: Response to phenelzine and amitriptyline in subtypes of outpatient depression. *Archives of General Psychiatry*, 39: 1041–1049, 1982.
4. Price, L. H., Connell, Y., and Nelson, J. D.: Lithium augmentation of combined neuroleptic therapy: Tricyclic treatment of delusional depression. *American Journal of Psychiatry*, 140: 318–322, 1983.
5. DeMontigery, D., Grunberg, F., Mayer, A., and Deschenes, J.-P.: Lithium induces rapid relief of depression in tricyclic antidepressant non-responders. *British Journal of Psychiatry*, 138: 252–256, 1981.
6. Ross, D. R., Walker, J. I., and Peterson, J.: Akathisia induced by amoxapine. *American Journal of Psychiatry*, 140: 115–116, 1983.
7. Anton, R. and Sexauer, J. D.: Efficacy of amoxapine in psychotic depression. *American Journal of Psychiatry*, 140: 1344–1347, 1983.
8. Sheehan, D. V., Claycomb, J. B., and Kouretas, M.: Monoamine oxidase inhibitors: Prescription and patient management. *International Journal of Psychiatric Medicine*, 10: 99–121, 1980–81.

CASE 19: ANTIDEPRESSANT-INDUCED SIDE EFFECTS

A 68-year-old man with a long history of recurrent depression presents for treatment at a local university-hospital-affiliated psychiatric outpatient clinic. The patient has no known significant medical problems. However, trials of a variety of antidepressant drugs subsequently lead to a series of unfortunate side effects. Initially, the patient is given a trial of imipramine at a dose of 100 mg per day and within 2 days he develops dizziness and faints upon standing up.

1. Which drug is most indicated in a patient who has developed orthostatic hypotension:
   A. Nortriptyline
   B. Desipramine

C. Trazodone
D. Doxepin
E. Maprotiline
F. Phenelzine

Discussion

Orthostatic hypotension is a serious problem for elderly patients receiving tricyclic antidepressants. Nortriptyline appears to have few hypotensive effects. Like nortriptyline, the newer antidepressants nomifensine, and bupropion also have few hypotensive effects. Amitriptyline, imipramine, and desipramine can all cause hypotension, as can trazodone. Similarly, monoamine oxidase inhibitors such as tranylcypromine and phenelzine can cause serious hypotension.

Case Continued: The patient is put on trazodone and promptly becomes oversedated.

2. A drug that is relatively nonsedative is:
   A. Maprotiline
   B. Amitriptyline
   C. Desipramine
   D. Doxepin
   E. Nomifensine
   F. A and C
   G. C and E

Discussion

Of the conventional antidepressants, desipramine is probably the least sedating. Of the new antidepressants, bupropion and nomifensine are nonsedating and somewhat activating.

Case Continued: The patient mentions that he had been put on amitriptyline with good results 10 years previously. For that reason, he is started on amitriptyline with a dosage escalation to 150 mg per day over a 1-week period. The patient promptly goes into urinary retention and becomes simultaneously confused.

3. Of the conventional and new antidepressants, the drug with the fewest anticholinergic effects is:
   A. Desipramine
   B. Amoxapine
   C. Trazodone
   D. Maprotiline

Discussion

The decision about which antidepressant drug has the fewest anticholinergic side effects is often relevant in the treatment of elderly patients. Anticholinergic effects can cause a central confusional syndrome which, at worst, resembles an atropine psychosis. In addition, exacerbations of closed-angle glaucoma, paralytic ileus, parotitis, and urinary obstruction, especially in patients with benign prostatic hypertrophy, may occur as serious manifestations of anticholinergic toxicity. Although desipramine, maprotiline, and amoxapine have all been reported to have relatively few anticholinergic side effects as compared to amitriptyline, doxepin, and protriptyline, all of these agents have anticholinergic effects, especially when given in full clinical dosages. Trazodone is unique in that it truly does not appear to have anticholinergic effects.

Answers

1. (A)
2. (G)
3. (C)

References

1. Glassman, A. H. and Bigger, J. T.: Cardiovascular effects of therapeutic doses of tricyclic antidepressants: A review. *Archives of General Psychiatry*, 38: 815–820, 1981.
2. Roose, S. P., Glassman, A., Siris, S. G., *et al.*: Comparison of imipramine- and nortriptyline-induced orthostatic hypotension: A meaningful difference. *Journal of Clinical Psychopharmacology*, 1: 316–319, 1981.

3. Hayes, J. R., Bonn, G. F., and Rosenbaum, A. H.: Incidence of orthostatic hypotension in patients with primary affective disorders treated with tricyclic antidepressants. *Mayo Clinic Proceedings*, 52: 509–512, 1977.
4. Glassman, A. H., Bigger, J. T., Giardina, E. V., *et al.*: Clinical characteristics of imipramine-induced orthostatic hypotension. *Lancet*, 1: 468–472, 1979.
5. Ayd, F.: New antidepressant drugs. *Psychiatric Annals*, 11: 11–17, 1981.
6. Steele, T. E.: Adverse reactions suggesting amoxapine-induced dopamine blockade. *American Journal of Psychiatry*, 139: 1500–1501, 1982.
7. Giardina, E. G. V. and Bigger, J. T.: Antiarrhythmic effect of imipramine hydrochloride in patients with ventricular premature complexes without psychological depression. *American Journal of Cardiology*, 50: 162–179, 1982.
8. Bigger, J. T., Kantor, S. J., Glassman, A. H., and Perel, J. M.: Cardiovascular effects of tricyclic antidepressants. In: *Psychopharmacology: A Generation of Progress* (eds.: M. A. Lipton, A. DiMascio, and K. F. Killam). Raven Press, New York, 1978, pp. 1033–1046.
9. Davidson, J. and Wenger, T.: When and how to use antidepressants in patients with cardiovascular disease. *Drug Therapy*, 12: 55, 1982.

CASE 20: USE OF NEWER ANTIDEPRESSANTS

A 38-year-old man has an 8-month history of symptoms compatible with a major depressive disorder. He has periods of sadness, feelings of worthlessness, hopelessness, and helplessness, lack of energy, and lack of motivation. In addition, the patient has a history of early-morning awakening, at which time he generally worries excessively. The patient has a physical examination, which yields essentially normal results with the exception of an occasional premature ventricular contraction. The patient states that he is willing to be treated with an antidepressant, but expresses fear of being "poisoned" by the medication.

1. The drug most likely to suppress the patient's premature ventricular contractions is:
   A. Desipramine
   B. Trazodone
   C. Doxepin
   D. Methylphenidate
2. The drug likely to increase this patient's premature ventricular contractions is:

A. Maprotiline
B. Bupropion
C. Trazodone
D. Amoxapine

Discussion

Most conventional and some of the newer antidepressants, including desipramine, have quinidine-like effects that can suppress ventricular irritability, including premature ventricular contractions. Trazodone appears to have relatively less quinidine-like effects, and thus is less likely to suppress such contractions. Conversely, there is some evidence that trazodone may actually increase the frequency of premature ventricular contractions. Finally, desipramine, which has quinidine-like effects, can increase these contractions in patients with mitral-valve prolapse.

3. Which of the following newer antidepressants appears to be most seizure-inducing:
   A. Trazodone
   B. Maprotiline
   C. Amoxapine
   D. Bupropion
   E. Nomifensine
4. Which of the following drugs is least toxic in an overdose:
   A. Maprotiline
   B. Amoxapine
   C. Trazodone
   D. Nomifensine
   E. Bupropion
   F. A, B, and C
   G. C, D, and E
5. The drug with the least anticholinergic effects is:
   A. Maprotiline
   B. Amoxapine
   C. Trazodone
6. The most prevalent side effect of trazodone is:
   A. Sedation

B. Anticholinergic effects
C. Cardiac effects
D. Hypotension

Discussion

Over the past 4 years, a number of new antidepressants have come on the market. Each has been featured as having advantages over the conventional antidepressants, and each has been shown in clinical practice to have specific disadvantages. Although, as with the conventional antidepressants, a new antidepressant may be specifically efficacious in a given patient, the overall efficacies of the new drugs are generally equal. With respect to disadvantages, maprotiline appears especially prone to cause seizures. Amoxapine has dopamine-blocking properties and can cause parkinsonian symptoms and tardive dyskinesia, and trazodone and maprotiline are especially sedating. Also, amoxapine and maprotiline are especially toxic in an overdose. With respect to advantages, trazodone appears especially safe in an overdose, and has few if any anticholinergic effects. Amoxapine and possibly trazodone may have a rapid onset of action.

Answers

1. (A)
2. (C)
3. (B)
4. (G)
5. (C)
6. (A)

References

1. Alexopoulos, G. S. and Shamoian, C. A.: Tricyclic antidepressants and cardiac patients with pacemakers. *American Journal of Psychiatry*, 139(4): 519–520, 1982.
2. Pariser, S. F., Reynolds, J. C., Falko, J. M., Jones, B., and Mencer, D. L.: Arrhythmia induced by a tricyclic antidepressant in a patient with undiagnosed mitral valve prolapse. *American Journal of Psychiatry*, 138(4): 522–523, 1981.

3. Richelson, E.: Pharmacology of antidepressants in use in the United States. *Journal of Clinical Psychiatry*, 43(11): 4–11, 1982.
4. Janowsky, D. S., Curtis, G., Zisook, S., *et al.*: Ventricular arrhythmias possibly aggravated by trazodone. *American Journal of Psychiatry*, 140: 796–797, 1983.
5. Veith, R. C., Raskind, M. A., Caldwell, J. H., *et al.*: Cardiovascular effects of tricyclic antidepressants in depressed patients with chronic heart disease. *New England Journal of Medicine*, 306: 954–959, 1982.
6. Ross, D. R., Walker, J. I., and Peterson, J.: Akathisia induced by amoxapine. *American Journal of Psychiatry*, 140: 115–116, 1983.
7. Ayd, F.: New antidepressant drugs. *Psychiatric Annals*, 11: 11–17, 1981.

CASE 21: TREATMENT OF A CASE OF MANIA WITH LITHIUM AND OTHER ANTIMANIC DRUGS

Judith E. is a 32-year-old unmarried, white, unemployed woman secretary with a 10-year history of intermittant manic and depressive episodes. Between each of these she has been essentially euthymic. The episodes have occurred with increasing frequency over the years, and recently as often as twice per year. More often than not they were manic episodes, but depressive episodes occurred approximately one in three times. The episodes lasted approximately 2 months. The patient was brought to the university hospital emergency room displaying increased speech, irritability, euphoria, grandiosity, and a recent history of planning to set up a transcontinental telegraph business, to which end she had approached members of the New York Stock Exchange. She had been making numerous long-distance phone calls, overspending money, and sleeping approximately 2 hours per night. Her symptoms had begun approximately 2 weeks earlier at which time she had been faced with having to take a job that she considered demeaning. At the time of her initial examination the patient was dressed brightly in a red-and-magenta muu-muu. She spoke rapidly about her numerous contacts and business dealings and showed euphoria, except when confronted about details of these dealings, at which time she became irritable. She showed flight of ideas, and answered that since moving to this city 2 months ago she had stopped taking her lithium. She said she had been lonely and depressed since moving until 2 weeks before her presentation, when everything started working out for her. A tentative diagnosis of bipolar disorder, manic phase, was made. Initially, it was felt that the patient might be able to be managed as an outpatient, but during the closing part of the interview she began to insist that she did not need medication, since she was doing so well. Hospitalization was suggested, and after initially resisting, the patient agreed, saying she wanted "to help those poor souls on the psychiatric unit." During the first 2 days of her hospitalization, the patient continued to be verbomanic, grandiose, and mildy euphoric. She also was extremely manipulative, categorizing the staff into those who thought that she was sane and charming and those who felt she was conniving and a fraud. She showed a remarkable tendency to talk about the deficiencies of the inpatient unit and its personnel.

1. For a patient such as this, the initial pharmacologic treatment(s) of choice would be:
   A. Haloperidol
   B. Carbamazepine
   C. Lithium carbonate
   D. Lithium carbonate plus haloperidol
   E. Lithium carbonate plus carbamazepine
2. Blood for measurement of the serum lithium level should be drawn as follows:
   A. 1 hour after the last lithium dose
   B. 12 hours after the last lithium dose
   C. 24 hours after the last lithium dose
3. The optimal serum lithium level for an acutely manic patient is:
   A. 0.5 to 0.8 mEq/liter
   B. 0.8 to 1.1 mEq/liter
   C. 1.1 to 1.4 mEq/liter
   D. 1.4 to 1.8 mEq/liter

Case Continued: On the third day of her hospitalization in a regimen of thrice weekly group and individual psychotherapy, the patient was begun on a trial of lithium carbonate. Lithium was started at a dose of 300 mg, b.i.d. for 4 days. On the fourth day of lithium administration, a serum specimen taken 12 hours after the preceeding night's dose showed a level of 0.4 mEq/liter. Since an eventual level of 1.2 mEq/liter was targeted, the lithium dose was increased to 300 mg q.i.d. for 3 days, at which time the serum level was 0.9 mEq/liter. An additional increase to 600 mg, t.i.d. led to a serum level of 1.1 mEq/liter 3 days later. By the twelfth hospital day, the patient was slightly improved with respect to her grandiose ideas. She no longer talked incessantly about her telegraph business, and was less irritable. She was still verbomanic and showed mild flight of ideas.

Discussion

At this time, the use of lithium is the treatment of choice for mania and hypomania, as well as for the prophylaxis of future manic and depressive episodes. Since lithium may take from 1 to 3 weeks to be effective, the short-term use of an antipsychotic drug may help in decreasing manic symptoms until the lithium takes effect, but only if it is needed should it be used. In the case described, the patient's behavior was mild enough to warrant using lithium alone.

Case Continued: On the sixteenth hospital day, a serum lithium level of 1.2 mEq/liter was obtained, with the patient continuing to receive lithium 600 mg, t.i.d. At that time she was beginning to complain of frequent urination, and was observed to be using the water fountain frequently. Furthermore, she had developed a fine tremor of her hands, which she disliked having.

4. The most frequent complaint of patients with bipolar affective disorders who are receiving lithium is:
   A. Mental dulling
   B. Dry mouth
   C. Frequent urination
   D. Tremor of the hands
   E. Missing the highs of mania

Discussion

Although lithium is often an effective prophylactic agent for bipolar disorder producing a decrease in the frequency and intensity of episodes, patients with bipolar disorders are often noncompliant. The patient often states that he or she misses the high of mania, and the natural denial occurring with a hypomanic state may cause the patient to be overconfident. For this reason, it is extremely important that the patient have an ongoing therapeutic relationship, and that the tendency to stop medications be done with continuing psychotherapeutic support.

5. The best pharmacologic treatment for lithium-induced tremor is:
   A. Diazepam
   B. Chlorpromazine
   C. Propranolol
   D. Imipramine
   E. None of the above

Discussion

The side effects of lithium may be bothersome, and are a major cause of therapeutic noncompliance with this drug. Among the side effects that are frequent are tremor and a diabetes-insipidus-like syndrome. Both these symptoms are at least partially responsive to decreasing the lithium dose, and the lithium tremor is treatable with a beta-adrenergic blocking agent such as propranolol.

Case Continued: By the twentieth hospital day, the patient was only very mildly hypomanic. She was no longer manipulative, had been elected to be the community-meeting president on her ward, and was now well liked by the nursing staff. Since she had improved, and since her serum lithium level had now increased to 1.4mEq/liter, it was decided to decrease her lithium dosage to one 300-mg tablet, q.i.d. Four days later, her serum lithium level was 1.0 mEq/liter. At this dose, the patient's tremor became minimal, and her diabetes insipidus syndrome disappeared.

6. When bipolar affective disorder patients receiving lithium become depressed, their serum lithium levels generally:
   A. Increase
   B. Decrease
   C. Stay the same
7. The implication of an increasing lithium level is that:
   A. The patient will fall out of the therapeutic range

B. The lithium may cause toxicity
C. There are no clinical implications

Discussion

For unknown reasons, larger amounts of lithium are required to maintain a given serum level when a patient is manic than when the same patient is depressed. Therefore, as a patient's mania remits, a reduction in lithium dosage may be necessary to avoid an increase in the serum level of the drug that puts it into the toxic range. In addition, serum lithium levels of 1.1 to 1.5 mEq/liter are usually necessary to treat acute mania, while lithium levels of only 0.8 to 1.0 mEq/liter are necessary to maintain prophylaxis.

Case Continued: The patient began to speak of wanting to leave the hospital and to return home. Dispositional planning occurred, with the patient meeting twice with her designated outpatient therapist before discharge, which occurred on the twenty-eighth hospital day. The unit social worker worked with the patient to help her seek employment, as well as to smooth the transition back to her apartment. At discharge the patient's lithium level was 0.9 mEq/liter. She was quite gregarious and cheerful, but showed none of her previous grandiosity or verbomania.

Answers

1. (C)
2. (B)
3. (C)
4. (E)
5. (C)
6. (A)
7. (B)

References

1. Prien, R. F., Klett, C. J., Caffey, E. M., Jr.: Lithium carbonate and imipramine in prevention of affective episodes. *Archives of General Psychiatry*, 29: 420–425, 1973.
2. Cooper, T. B., Gershon, S., Kline, N., and Schou, M.: *Lithium: Controversies and Unresolved Issues*. Excerpta Medica, Amsterdam, 1979.

3. Peselow, E. D., Dunner, D. L., Fieve, R. R., and Lautin, A.: Lithium carbonate and weight gain. *Journal of Affective Disorders*, 2: 303–310, 1980.
4. Vestergaard, P., Amdisen, A., and Schou, M.: Clinically significant side effects of lithium treatment: A survey of 232 patients in long term treatment. *Acta Psychiatrica Scandinavica*, 62: 193–200, 1980.
5. Tosteson, D. C.: Lithium and mania. *Scientific American*, 244: 164–174, 1981.
6. Tyrer, S. and Shopsin, B.: Neural and neuromuscular side-effects of lithium. In: *Handbook of Lithium Therapy* (ed.: F. N. Johnson). University Park Press, Baltimore, 1980, pp. 289–322.
7. Amdisen, A. and Andersen, C. J.: Lithium treatment and thyroid function: A function of 237 patients in long-term lithium treatment. *Pharmacopsychiatry*, 15: 149–155, 1982.
8. Gaby, N. S., Lefkowitz, D. S., and Israel, J. R.: Treatment of lithium tremor with metoprolol. *American Journal of Psychiatry*, 140: 593–595, 1983.
9. Roose, S. P., Nornberger, J. I., Dunner, D. L., Blood, D. K., and Fieve, R. R.: Cardiac sinus node dysfunction during lithium treatment. *American Journal of Psychiatry*, 130: 804–806, 1979.

CASE 22: MAINTENANCE DRUG THERAPY IN A PATIENT WITH AFFECTIVE DISORDER

A 52-year-old white male businessman has recently moved to the area. He contacts your office for an appointment. He explains that he was recently released from the hospital following treatment of his third "nervous breakdown." He states that he has been told by his doctors that he has manic–depressive illness, depressed type. He begins to explain his past difficulties. His most recent "breakdown" occurred while he was gainfully employed. The "breakdown" was characterized by depression, with multiple vegetative symptoms, including weight loss and insomnia, loss of interest, and preoccupation with morbid thoughts. He relates that he had a similar depressive episode 2 years previously and had a manic-type illness 20 years previously. He states that his manic episode caused him the greatest hardship, leading to his being fired by a prestigious company and resulting in a long-term hospitalization at a state hospital. You inquire which medications he is receiving, and he states that he is currently taking imipramine (Tofranil) 150 mg at bedtime and lithium carbonate 600 mg in the morning and at bedtime. He relates that he was discharged from the hospital approximately 1 month previously, and would like you to be his doctor. He has recently acquired a job and is worried about the possibility of having another "breakdown," which would jeopardize his career. He asks about the need for medications and the length of time that he will be taking the medications.

1. The natural history of bipolar illness demonstrates that one can expect an average time until relapse in patients not receiving prophylactic medications (lithium carbonate or carbamazepine) of:
   A. 4 months
   B. 8 months
   C. 12 months
   D. 16 months
2. Of patients receiving lithium carbonate on a maintenance basis, who have documented manic–depressive illness, a relapse occurs on the average of every:
   A. 8 months
   B. 16 months
   C. 32 months
   D. 72 months

Discussion

Early studies of the prophylactic value of lithium carbonate, done by Baastrup and Schou, established the efficacy and importance of long-term maintenance lithium treatment in bipolar manic illness. It is therefore of great importance to consider this information in the long-term treatment of patients with bipolar illness. A patient such as is illustrated by this case, who presents with three documented episodes typical of bipolar affective disorder, occuring at a time in his life when another psychotic breakdown could be extremely damaging, would best be put on long-term maintenance lithium carbonate therapy.

3. When a group of patients with a diagnosis of bipolar disorder is put on placebo, and compared with a second group receiving maintenance lithium therapy, the percentage of placebo-receiving patients who relapse after 5 months will be approximately:
   A. 0%
   B. 25%
   C. 50%

D. 75%
E. 100%

4. The percentage of patients with bipolar disorders who are given lithium and who will relapse after 5 months will be approximately:
   A. 0%
   B. 25%
   C. 50%
   D. 75%
   E. 100%

Discussion

Although Baastrap and Schou first suggested that almost all of their patients who were maintained on lithium carbonate were protected from relapse, subsequent studies, as outlined in the excellent review by Davis, have shown that approximately 36% of patients with affective disorder receiving lithium maintenance therapy do relapse, while 79% of patients receiving placebo relapse.

5. In comparing the prophylactic effect of lithium carbonate in unipolar (motor depressive disorder) versus bipolar patients, a better prophylactic effect was observed in the group of:
   A. Unipolar patients (major depressive disorder)
   B. Bipolar patients

Discussion

One might expect that a patient with bipolar affective illness will be most responsive to lithium carbonate, since lithium is the drug of choice in manic as opposed to depressive episodes. Prophylactic studies, however, have shown that patients with unipolar affective disorders who have been adequately treated for their depression and are then given on lithium carbonate maintenance therapy in fact show a slightly better prophylactic effect than patients in the bipolar group.

6. In patients who have typical bipolar disorder or schizoaffective disorder, the following is considered true:

A. Studies have shown that the number of affective episodes requiring hospitalization decreases with lithium carbonate maintenance therapy
B. The total number of months spent in the hospital of patients receiving lithium carbonate therapy is shortened
C. Some schizoprhenic patients develop lithium-induced central nervous system toxicity
D. All of the above

Discussion

A number of studies have pointed toward the possible efficacy of lithium carbonate in patients with atypical affective disorders, and in subtypes of affective illness in which schizophrenic features are present. Studies have shown that in patients with prominent affective symptoms, the number of hospitalizations decreases during lithium carbonate therapy. In addition, the episodes, when they do occur, are less lengthy. In some cases, however, schizophrenic patients have been shown to develop a toxic picture, with worsening of their mental status following lithium carbonate administration. One should use lithium carbonate carefully, and be aware of possible toxicity.

7. The following statements about combining lithium carbonate and antidepressant drugs are true:
   A. Monoamine oxidase inhibitors (MAOIs) and lithium carbonate can be used together without adverse interactions
   B. Tricyclic antidepressants and lithium carbonate have been shown to have a good therapeutic effect when used together
   C. Monoamine oxidase inhibitors and lithium carbonate have been shown to have good therapeutic effect when used together
   D. All of the above

Discussion

Patients who have been maintained on lithium carbonate and who show a recurrence of affective symptoms, such as depression, warrant addition of tricyclic antidepressants or MAOIs. Antidepressant drugs and lithium, given together, have been shown to have good therapeutic effects, and there have been no specific adverse interactions other than the expected potential side effects of each separate drug. With some patient subtypes there has been the suggestion that lithium combined with a tricyclic antidepressant may be slightly more effective than use of a tricyclic antidepressant alone. There have also been suggestions that MAOIs may become more effective in treatment-resistant patients when lithium is added. Polypharmacy, however, should be discouraged unless there is a clear-cut indication for it and careful assessment of the potential side effects of each drug individually. It is helpful, when using more than one drug, to start one drug at a time, carefully monitoring its side effects.

8. The subtype of bipolar disorder that has been shown to respond least well to lithium carbonate is:
   A. A very rapidly cycling illness with four or more affective episodes per year
   B. An illness with only manic episodes
   C. An illness with affective episodes occurring very infrequently, such as once every 10 years
   D. All of the above

Discussion

Studies have suggested that rapidly cycling bipolar disorders may represent a severe form of bipolar illness. Patients in this group have been shown to have relatively less impressive responses to lithium carbonate.

9. Side effects associated with lithium carbonate maintenance therapy may include:
   A. Lowering of the level of serum-protein-bound iodine
   B. Polyvria
   C. Confusion
   D. Tremor
   E. All of the above
10. Lithium carbonate can produce abnormal thyroid indices in as many as 20% of patients at some time during treatment:
   A. True
   B. False

11. The most common thyroid test(s) used to follow thyroid function in patients in lithium carbonate should include:
    A. T3
    B. T4
    C. Palpation of the thyroid
    D. All of the above

Discussion

Abnormal thyroid indices, occurring at some time during treatment are common in patients receiving lithium carbonate maintenance therapy. The most common problem is goiter formation, and the induction of a hypothyroid state which, although commonly mentioned, is relatively rare. Careful follow-up of patients receiving lithium carbonate maintenance therapy should include periodic thyroid tests and palpation of the thyroid for enlargement or goiter formation. An internist should be consulted if thyroid problems develop. Supplemental thyroid medication is indicated if lithium is to be continued. Patients may, with only a single dose of lithium carbonate, develop polyuria. This is considered to be a diabetes-insipidus-like syndrome, mediated by a vasopressin-sensitive adenyl cyclase in the kidney. The possibility of actual kidney deterioration and impairment of renal function is, however, extremely low during lithium carbonate therapy. Tremor and central nervous system symptoms, such as confusion, are signs of severe lithium toxicity, and all patients should be carefully educated, as should their families about the possibility of these side effects. Propranolol or metoprolol has been suggested by some clinicians as effective in counteracting lithium carbonate-induced tremor. Metoprolol may have an advantage over propranolol in being less likely to precipitate depression. Low doses of diazepam (Valium) may also be helpful in some patients in treating lithium tremor. Some geriatric patients are especially susceptible to the side effects of lithium on the central nervous system at lower than expected serum levels of this drug.

12. Patients who have been receiving lithium carbonate for 10 to 15 years have shown tardive dyskinesias similar to those caused by the phenothiazines:
    A. True
    B. False

Discussion

Long-term maintenance therapy with lithium carbonate suggests that the patient is always at risk for acute side effects, but chronic difficulties such as those found with the phenothiazines have not been well documented.

13. The expected percentage of patients with a history of depression who were previously treated with ECT and who relapse has been shown to be:
    A. 20%
    B. 40%
    C. 60%
    D. 90%
14. Patients treated with ECT who are then put on tricyclic-drug maintenance therapy show a relapse rate of:
    A. 20%
    B. 40%
    C. 60%
    D. 80%

Discussion

As clearly delineated in the review by Davis, and in the work of Seager and Bird, maintenance therapy with an antidepressant medication is indicated.

15. Tricyclic antidepressant drugs will occasionally precipitate mania in a patient with bipolar disease who is depressed:
    A. True
    B. False

Discussion

Caution in the use of tricyclic drugs is indicated in patients with documented bipolar illness. The patient represented in this case had clear-cut manic–depressive bipolar episodes, and maintenance therapy with a tricyclic drug could put the patient at risk for an exacerbation of the manic component of the illness. Once the depressive episode is successfully treated with an antidepressant, further management might be to administer lithium carbonate alone. Some investigators feel that lithium is clearly the prophylactic agent of choice in bipolar disease.

Answers

1. (B)
2. (D)
3. (C)
4. (B)
5. (A)
6. (D)
7. (D)
8. (A)
9. (E)
10. (A)
11. (D)
12. (B)
13. (C)
14. (B)
15. (A)

References

1. Baastrup, P. C. and Schou, M.: Lithium as a prophylactic agent against recurrent depressions and manic-depressive psychosis. *Archives of General Psychiatry*, 16: 162–172, 1967.
2. Baastrup, P. C. and Schou, M.: Prophylactic lithium. *Lancet*, 2: 349–350, 1968.
3. Baastrup, P. C. and Schou, M.: Prophylactic lithium. *Lancet*, 1: 1419–1422, 1968.
4. Davis, J. M.: Overview: Maintenance therapy in psychiatry: II. Affective disorders. *American Journal of Psychiatry*, 133: 1–13, 1976.
5. Perris, C.: A study of cycloid psychosis. *Acta Psychiatrica Scandinavica*, 50: 188, 1974.
6. Dunner, D. L. and Fieve, R. R.: Clinical factors in lithium carbonate prophylaxis failure. *Archives of General Psychiatry*, 30: 229–233, 1974.
7. Seager, C. P. and Bird, R. L.: Imipramine with electrical treatment in depression: A controlled trial. *Journal of Mental Sciences,* 108: 704–707, 1962.
8. Cooper, T. B., Gershon, S., Kline, N., and Schou, M.: *Lithium: Controversies and Unresolved Issues*. Excerpta Medica, Amsterdam, 1979.
9. Gaby, N. S., Lefkowitz, D. S., and Israel, J. R.: Treatment of lithium tremor with metoprolol. *American Journal of Psychiatry*, 140: 593–595, 1983.
10. Amdisen, A. and Andersen, C. J.: Lithium treatment and thyroid function: A survey of 237 patients in long-term lithium treatment. *Pharmacopsychiatry*, 15: 149–155, 1982.

11. Cowdry, R. W., Wehr, T. A., Zis, A. P., and Goodwin, F. K.: Thyroid abnormalities associated with rapid-cycling bipolar illness. *Archives of General Psychiatry*, 40: 414–419, 1983.
12. Peselow, E. D., Dunner, D. L., Fieve, R. R., and Lautin, A.: Lithium carbonate in weight gain. *Journal of Affective Disorders*, 2: 303–310, 1980.
13. Vestergaard, P., Amdisen, A., and Schou, M.: Clinically significant side effects of lithium treatment: A survey of 232 patients in long-term treatment. *Acta Psychiatrica Scandinavica*, 62: 193–200, 1980.
14. Thomsen, K.: Renal handling of lithium at non-toxic and toxic serum lithium levels. *Danish Medical Bulletin*, 25: 106–115, 1978.
15. Wallin, L., Alling, C., and Aurell, M.: Impairment of renal function in patients on long-term lithium treatment. *Clinical Nephrology*, 18: 23–28, 1982.
16. Lippman, S.: Is lithium bad for the kidneys? *Journal of Clinical Psychiatry*, 44: 220–225, 1982.
17. Janin, M. W.: Lithium prophylaxis of tricyclic antidepressant induced mania in bipolar patients. *American Journal of Psychiatry*, 139: 683, 1982.
18. Prien, R. F., Klett, C. J., and Caffey, E. M., Jr.: Lithium carbonate and imipramine in prevention of affective episodes. *Archives of General Psychiatry*, 29: 420, 1973.
19. Kane, J. M., Quitkin, F. M., Rifkin, A., *et al.*: Lithium carbonate and imipramine in the prophylaxis of unipolar and bipolar II illness. *Archives of General Psychiatry*, 39: 1065–1069, 1982.
20. Lapierre, Y. D.: Control of lithium tremor with propranolol. *Canadian Medical Association Journal*, 114: 619–624, 1976.
21. Dunner, D. L., Fleiss, J. L., and Fieve, R. R.: Lithium carbonate prophylaxis failure. *British Journal of Psychiatry*, 129: 40–44, 1976.

CASE 23: MAINTENANCE THERAPY WITH LITHIUM CARBONATE

Mr. O. is a 48-year-old Hispanic male with a 20-year history of bipolar mood swings. After his most recent affective episode, which was manic, the patient was followed in an outpatient clinic by a third-year psychiatric resident who treated him with a combination of insight-oriented psychotherapy, supportive psychotherapy, and lithium therapy. He was seen at weekly intervals for 4 months, with serum lithium levels being monitored twice monthly for 2 months and monthly thereafter. A dose of lithium 300 mg, q.i.d. yielded serum levels between 0.8 and 1.0 mEq/liter. The patient is currently sad and has a lack of energy.

1. The patient's symptoms of anergy and sadness may be due to:
   A. Bipolar depression
   B. Lithium-induced hypothyroidism
   C. Hypocalcemia
   D. Renal tubular fibrosis
   E. A and B
   F. B and D
2. A serious but infrequent effect of lithium therapy is:
   A. Cerebral arteriosclerosis
   B. Renal tubular fibrosis with azotemia
   C. Irreversible hypothyroidism
   D. None of the above

Case Continued: Since the patient had not had laboratory testing done since his hospitalization, a laboratory battery, including T3, T4, serum electrolytes, and serum creatinine was obtained to rule out any renal damage, lithium-induced hypothyroidism, or both. None of these tests was abnormal. Therefore, a depressive episode due to lithium-induced hypothyroidism having been ruled out, the patient was diagnosed as having developed a bipolar depressive episode.

3. The relative ability of lithium and tricyclic antidepressants such as imipramine to prevent the onset of depression in patients with bipolar illness is:
   A. Approximately equal
   B. Lithium is a much more effective prophylactic agent than are the tricyclic antidepressants
   C. Tricyclic antidepressants are much more effective prophylactic agents than lithium
   D. Because of its ability to induce a mood switch to mania, a tricyclic antidepressant is indicated

Discussion

Several studies have evaluated the ability of lithium and tricyclic antidepressants to prevent relapse in psychiatric patients with bipolar or unipolar, or both kinds of illness. Generally, at least in patients with bipolar illness, both lithium and the tricyclic antidepressants significantly and to an equal degree, decrease the relapse rate of depressive patients. In bipolar illness, lithium may be the indicated drug for the prophylaxis of depression, since the tricyclic antidepressants may cause a switch from depression to mania, or an increase in the frequency of manic–depressive cycles. There is some clinical evidence that in bipolar patients and in unipolar patients whose depression does not respond to, or is not effectively prevented by either lithium or a tricyclic antidepressant, a combination of lithium plus a tricyclic antidepressant, or the use of carbamazepine, alone or with lithium, may be efficacious.

4. A problem(s) coincident with giving a depressed patient who has a bipolar illness a conventional antidepressant drug is (are):
   A. The induction of rapid mood cycling
   B. The induction of a switch to mania
   C. The induction of a central anticholinergic syndrome
   D. All of the above
   E. None of the above

Case Continued: After a discussion of their side effects, including the risk of inducing a switch to mania or an increase in the frequency of cycling, the patient and therapist decided to begin a course of trimipramine. Trimipramine was begun in a dose of 50 mg daily, and increased over a period of 2 weeks to 200 mg per day, a clinically adequate dosage. The patient experienced mild sedation as well as a dry mouth and mild constipation from the trimipramine, but generally tolerated it well. After 3 weeks of receiving trimipramine he reported sleeping better, and by the sixth week he felt euthymic. The trimipramine was continued for one more month in full doses, and then tapered to cessation over a period of 2 weeks to prevent withdrawal symptoms due to "cholinergic overdrive." The patient did not experience a renewal of symptoms after stopping the trimipramine.

Discussion

The management of mood swings into depression presents several problems. Use of a tricyclic antidepressant or monoamine oxidase inhibitor (MAOI) carries the risk of inducing a manic episode, or of inducing a greater frequency of manic–depressive episodes. It is hoped that lithium will be effective enough to prevent serious future depressions, but this is not always the case. Since not infrequently a tricyclic antidepressant or MAOI may alleviate depression without causing mania or rapid mood cycling, a trial of antidepressant drug therapy is indicated along with lithium. Possibly, phenelzine (Nardil) is especially indicated. However, once the patient is euthymic, or becomes hypomanic, the antidepressant should be stopped, and lithium should be continued throughout the therapy. Ann antipsychotic drug may be useful in treating antidepressant-induced manic or hypomanic episodes, in conjunction with lithium.

Answers

1. (E)
2. (D)
3. (A)
4. (D)

References

1. Davis, J. M.: Overview: Maintenance therapy in psychiatry: II. Affective disorders. *American Journal of Psychiatry*, 133: 1, 1976.
2. Oppenheim, G.: Drug-induced rapid cycling: Possible outcomes and management. *American Journal of Psychiatry*, 139(7): 939–941, 1982.
3. Cowdry, R. W., Wehr, T. A., Ziz, A. P., and Goodwin, F. K.: Thyroid abnormalities associated with rapid-cycling bipolar illness. *Archives of General Psychiatry*, 40: 414–419, 1983.
4. Janin, M. W.: Lithium prophylaxis of tricyclic antidepressant induced mania in bipolar patients. *American Journal of Psychiatry*, 139: 683, 1982.
5. Plenge, P., Mellerup, E. T., and Bolwig, T. G.: Lithium treatment: Does the kidney prefer one daily dose instead of two? *Acta Psychiatrica Scandinavica*, 66: 121–128, 1982.
6. Cooper, T. B., Gershon, S., Kline, N., and Schou, M.: *Lithium: Controversies and Unresolved Issues*. Excerpta Medica, Amsterdam, 1979.
7. Prakash, R., Kelwala, S., and Ban, T. A.: Neurotoxicity with combined administration of lithium and a neuroleptic. *Comprehensive Psychiatry*, 23: 567–571, 1982.
8. Spring, G. and Frankel, M.: New data on lithium and haloperidol incompatibility. *American Journal of Psychiatry*, 138: 818–821, 1981.

9. Spring, G. K.: Neurotoxicity with combined use of lithium and thioridazine. *Journal of Clinical Psychiatry*, 40: 135–138, 1979.
10. Singh, S. V.: Lithium carbonate/fluphenazine decanoate producing irreversible brain damage. *Lancet*, 2: 278, 1982.

CASE 24: TREATMENT OF A MANIC PATIENT WITH CARBAMAZEPINE

The patient is a 32-year-old white male who has a long history of bipolar illness, consisting predominantly of manic interdispersed with depressive episodes. Previous treatment with adequate blood levels of lithium did not prove useful in alleviating the patient's manic symptoms. Haloperiodol did, however, decrease these symptoms, but there is worry that a tardive dyskinesia might develop.

1. A logical back-up drug for this patient is:
   A. Carbamazepine
   B. Oxazepam
   C. Imipramine
   D. Sodium pentothal
2. Drugs that have antimanic properties and that, if given over time, are preventive of manic and depressive episodes include:
   A. Haloperidol
   B. Carbamazepine
   C. Lithium carbonate
   D. Diazepam
   E. A and D
   F. B and C

Case Continued: The patient is taken off lithium for 1 week and is put on carbamazepine 200 mg per day. This dose is gradually increased over a period of 1 week. During the initial week of therapy, the patient complains of feeling dizzy.

3. The most dangerous side effect of carbamazepine is:
   A. Agranulocytosis
   B. Syncope

C. Nausea
D. Diarrhea
E. Confusion

4. The dose of carbamazepine should range from:
   A. 100 to 300 mg per day
   B. 200 to 400 mg per day
   C. 400 to 600 mg per day
   D. 600 to 1000 mg per day
5. Carbamazepine serum levels are useful in:
   A. Determining and monitoring toxicity
   B. Determining efficacy
   C. Determining at which dose agranulocytosis will occur
   D. Of no use at all

Case Continued: Over the next 3 weeks, while receiving doses of carbamazepine 800 mg per day the patient shows virtually no clinical improvement. Indeed, his manic symptoms increase slightly.

6. If neither lithium nor carbamazepine is individually useful in antagonizing manic symptoms:
   A. A combination of lithium and carbamazepine may be needed
   B. Addition of an antipsychotic drug may be necessary
   C. An immediate infusion of sodium valproate is indicated
   D. None of the above

Discussion

A number of studies have suggested that antipsychotic drugs, including haloperidol and lithium carbonate, are effective in the treatment of mania. There is also considerable evidence that carbamazepine and lithium have antimanic properties and exert a prophylactic effect against bipolar mood swings. Recently, European studies have indicated that sodium valproate has antimanic properties and antimanic and antidepressant prophylactic properties. There is little, if any, evidence that benzodiazepines, given in clinically acceptable doses, have antimanic effects. For patients with bipolar disorders who either show an inadequate response to lithium carbonate or are unable to tolerate the medication because of side effects, a trial of carbamazepine may be indicated. Although carbamazepine has been used most commonly in the treatment of temporal-lobe epilepsy and trigeminal neuralgia, patients who have bipolar illness without any evidence of abnormal brain electrical activity have been shown to respond beneficially to the drug. Carbamazepine has proved to be of use in a significant number of patients with mania who have not had a satisfactory response to lithium carbonate. Furthermore, there is evidence that a combination of lithium and carbamazepine may help nonresponders to either agent alone. Like lithium, carbamazepine appears to have antidepressant as well as antimanic properties, although this possibly needs to be more clearly documented. Since carbamazepine appears to have complex pharmacokinetic properties and has significant interactions with a variety of other drugs, it is important to monitor its serum levels on an ongoing basis. However, the specific serum level necessary for therapeutic benefit is not clear. Determining serum levels is useful in preventing toxicity. A dose range of 600 to 1,000 mg per day often yields an antimanic effect. Early concern over the possibility that the drug induced aplastic anemia appears to have been replaced by recognition that such events are exceedingly rare.

Answers

1. (A)
2. (F)
3. (A)
4. (D)
5. (A)
6. (A)

References

1. Ballenger, J. and Post, R.: Carbamazepine (Tegretol) in manic depressive illness: A new treatment. *American Journal of Psychiatry*, 137: 782–790, 1980.
2. Janin, M. W.: Lithium prophylaxis of tricyclic antidepressant induced mania in bipolar patients. *American Journal of Psychiatry*, 139: 683, 1982.
3. Post, R.: Carbamazepine's acute and prophylactic effect in manic and depressive illness: An update. *International Drug Therapy Newsletter*, 17: 2–3, 1982.
4. Okuma, R.: Therapeutic and prophylactic effects of carbamazepine in bipolar disorders. *Psychiatric Clinics of North America*, 6: 157–174, 1983.
5. Lipinski, J. E. and Pope, H. C.: Possible synergistic action between carba-

mazepine and lithium carbonate in the treatment of three acutely manic patients. *American Journal of Psychiatry*, 139: 948–949, 1982.
6. Chaudhry, R. P. and Waters, B. G.: Lithium and carbamazepine interaction: Possible neurotoxicity. *Journal of Clinical Psychiatry*, 44: 30–31, 1983.

CASE 25: LITHIUM CARBONATE AS AN ANTIDEPRESSANT

A 36-year-old man has a 10-year history of recurrent retarded depressions, between which he is creative and does well occupationally. Once, he had what appeared to be a hypomanic episode. He is now depressed and is hospitalized on an inpatient psychiatric unit for treatment of his depression.

1. It is likely that he would improve if he received:
   A. Lithium carbonate
   B. A monoamine oxidase inhibitor
   C. A tricyclic antidepressant
   D. Any of the above
2. Lithium carbonate is probably:
   A. Useful in treating "biologic" depression in patients with a history of bipolar manic–depressive illness
   B. Of no use in treating biologic depressions
   C. More effective than imipramine (Tofranil) in treating biologic depressions in bipolar patients
   D. A and C
   E. None of the above

Discussion

Lithium carbonate has been reported to have direct antidepressant effects in a number of studies. Although there is some disagreement over which subtypes of depression respond best to this drug, the general consensus is that manic–depressive patients who are depressed respond best to lithium carbonate. The serum level suggested ranges from 0.8 to 1.2 mEq/liter. One study, using a double-blind technique, has found lithium carbonate as effective as a tricyclic antidepressant.

Answers

1. (D)
2. (A)

References

1. Davis, J. M., Janowsky, D. S., and El-Yousef, M. K.: The use of lithium in clinical psychiatry. *Psychiatric Annals*, 3(2): 78–99, 1973.
2. DeMontigery, C., Grunberg, F., Mayer, A., and Deschenes, J.-P.: Lithium induces rapid relief of depression in tricyclic antidepressant drug non-responders. *British Journal of Psychiatry*, 138: 252–256, 1981.
3. Mendlewicz, J., Fieve, R. R., and Stallone, F.: Relationship between the effectiveness of lithium therapy and family history. *American Journal of Psychiatry*, 130: 1011–1013, 1973.

CASE 26: TREATMENT OF SCHIZOPHRENIFORM DISORDER

A 22-year-old man is brought to the emergency room by the police after walking on the beach naked at 6:00 A.M. and stating that he has been communing with God. There is no past psychiatric history. A mental-status examination shows the patient to be confused and disoriented as to time, place, and person. He believes he has been taken over by another being who is using him as part of a religious rite. This idea came to him over the past week, and caused him to walk off his job as a gasoline station attendant, at which he had been working for the last 2 years. He felt that the station operator was part of the plot to control him. The patient's mood is basically euphoric, he shows no insight into his delusions. There appear to be auditory hallucinations. He shows pressure of speech.

1. Correct statements about such a patient, who might be labeled as having a schizophreniform reaction, include:
   A. About 50% of patients labeled as having a schizophreniform disorder fulfill research criteria for the diagnosis of mania
   B. The prognosis for the present episode in such a patient may be quite good

C. Confusion often is a good prognostic sign in such patients
D. Such patients are likely to show a strong family history of schizophrenia

2. The differential diagnosis of the patient should include the following possibilities:
A. Schizophrenia, paranoid type
B. Bipolar disease, manic type
C. Organic brain syndrome due to hallucinogen ingestion
D. Amphetamine psychosis
E. All of the above

Discussion

Bipolar disorder, manic type; schizophrenia, paranoid type; amphetamine psychosis; and organic brain syndrome due to hallucinogens have many similarities. Historical data concerning the present illness, including its time of onset, duration, and contributing factors, and any previous history of emotional illness are critical in helping reach the specific diagnosis. A history of complete remissions between episodes favors bipolar illness. A history of drug ingestion supports the diagnosis of an organic brain syndrome due to hallucinogens, or amphetamine psychosis. Drug-induced states are more commonly marked by visual hallucinations and bizzare delusions than are schizophrenic syndromes or bipolar illness, but this differentiation is not absolute.

3. In addition to being useful in bipolar illness, manic type, lithium carbonate has been shown to be an effective prophylactic agent in the following illness:
A. Amphetamine psychosis
B. Organic brain syndrome
C. Schizoaffective disorder
D. Involutional melancholia
E. None of the above

4. The term "good-prognosis schizophrenia" is used to label patients who show a good chance of recovery, as opposed to those who proceed to chronicity. The following factors delineate this group:

A. Acute onset
B. Clouded sensorium
C. Good premorbid adjustment
D. Family history of affective disorder
E. All of the above

Discussion

Some authors feel that schizoaffective disorder is a diagnostic label without a disease. This syndrome has received a number of different labels in the past, including schizoaffective schizophrenia, reactive schizophrenia, schizophreniform psychosis, oneirophrenia, acute exhaustive psychosis, and remitting schizophrenia. When one carefully examines the diagnosis, based on research criteria, of patients who were diagnosed as having schizophreniform disorder, approximately half may receive a research diagnosis of mania. This diagnostic category has also been called "good-prognosis schizophrenia." This supposedly represents a subset of schizophrenic patients who have the good prognostic signs of acute onset, a clouded sensorium, good premorbid adjustment, precipitating factors, and a family history of affective disorder. As mentioned above, this disorder may actually be mania. The prognosis for these patients may be quite good.

5. Correct statements about the treatment of schizoaffective patients include:
   A. These patients almost never respond to lithium
   B. These patients almost never respond to electroconvulsive therapy
   C. The chances of the patient improving significantly without drug treatment are small
   D. These patients often respond to major tranquilizers

Discussion

Because patients carrying the diagnosis of schizophreniform disorder are probably a heterogeneous group, their response to any particular treatment awaits accurate diagnostic evaluation. However, it appears that a major subgroup of patients with such illness are suffering from an affective disorder, and will respond to lithium, electroconvulsive therapy, or major tranquilizers. One difficulty in evaluating treatment efficacy is that these patients not infrequently improve spontaneously.

6. Correct statements about the relative effectiveness of various treatments for acute-onset psychosis include:
   A. Lithium is better than major tranquilizers
   B. A combination of an activating and inactivating major tranquilizer is superior to lithium alone
   C. On a comparative basis, lithium carbonate, electroconvulsive therapy, and antipsychotic agents are generally equally effective
   D. Sedation with hypnotics is the treatment of choice

Discussion

Taylor *et al.* examined 26 consecutive patients with a diagnosis of acute schizophrenia upon admission to the psychiatric unit of a municipal hospital. The diagnoses were evaluated using research diagnostic criteria. The authors concluded that many patients receiving a diagnosis of acute schizophrenia actually had affective illness, and rarely satisfied rigorous diagnostic criteria for schizophrenia. In an earlier study, the clinical picture and response to treatment of 52 patients with an admission diagnosis of "acute schizophrenia" was investigated. These patients received their doctor's choice of treatment, and 90% showed marked improvement or full remission (including 15 of 17 who were given lithium alone). The authors concluded that the specific type of treatment—be it lithium, antipsychotic drugs, a combination of drugs, or electroconvulsive therapy, did not affect the case outcome.

7. Correct statements about the use of lithium in acute schizophrenic reactions include:
   A. A controlled study has indicated that lithium may be effective in preventing further attacks of this disorder
   B. The average lithium dosage would probably be between 300 and 600 mg, t.i.d.
   C. Severe side effects are not likely to occur with lithium blood levels below 1.0 mEq/liter

D. Lithium carbonate is the only effective lithium salt in the treatment of an acute schizophrenic reaction

Discussion

Due to a lack of controlled studies of different treatments, the specific treatment for acute schizophrenia or schizophreniform disorder is unknown. Probably because one is often dealing with an affective disorder, lithium has been shown to be effective. One controlled study utilized lithium carbonate in doses of 300 to 600 mg t.i.d. with resulting blood levels of approximately 1.0 mEq/liter. The researchers concluded that lithium was effective in preventing further attacks of the schizoaffective psychoses.

Answers

1. (A, B, and C)
2. (E)
3. (C)
4. (E)
5. (D)
6. (C)
7. (A, B, and C)

References

1. Taylor, M. A., Gaxtanga, P., and Abrams, R.: Manic-depressive illness and acute schizophrenia: A clinical, family history, and treatment-response study. *American Journal of Psychiatry*, 131: 678–682, 1974.
2. Robins, E. and Guze, S. B.: Establishment of diagnostic validity in psychiatric illness: Its application to schizophrenia. *American Journal of Psychiatry*, 126: 983–987, 1970.
3. Goodwin, D. W., Alderson, P., and Rosenthal, R.: Clinical significance of hallucinations in psychiatric disorders. *Archives of General Psychiatry*, 24: 76–80, 1971.
4. Smulevitch, A. B., Zavidovskaya, G. I., Igonin, A. L., Mikhailova, N. M.: The effectiveness of lithium in affective and schizoaffective psychoses. *British Journal of Psychiatry*, 125: 65–72, 1974.
5. Hirschowitz, J., Casper, R., Garver, D. L., and Chang, S.: Lithium response in good prognosis schizophrenia. *American Journal of Psychiatry*, 137: 915–920, 1980.

6. Price, L. H., Connell, Y., and Nelson, J. C.: Lithium augmentation of combined neuroleptic–tricyclic treatment of delusional depression. *American Journal of Psychiatry*, 140: 318–322, 1983.

CASE 27: DIAGNOSIS AND TREATMENT OF ACUTE MANIA

A 28-year-old male physician presents with irritability, euphoria, flight of ideas, grandiose ideas, logorrhea, insomnia, a history of overspending, increased energy, and calling strangers long distance all over the world and reversing the charges. These symptoms have occurred twice previously. Usually the patient functions very well, but he is prone to have spells of feeling pessimistic, worthless, useless, anergic, and sad. His mother is mentally healthy. His father committed suicide when the patient was 3 years old.

1. The most likely diagnosis of this patient is:
   A. Schizophrenia
   B. Passive–aggressive character disorder
   C. Alcoholism
   D. Bipolar disorder, manic type
2. The most efficacious drug for rapidly relieving the patient's symptoms is:
   A. An antipsychotic agent such as haloperidol (Haldol) or chlorpromazine (Thorazine)
   B. Lithium carbonate
   C. Chlordiazepoxide (Librium)
   D. A tricyclic antidepressant such as imipramine (Tofranil)
3. The most efficacious drug for relieving the patient's symptoms over a 2- to 3-week period is:
   A. An antipsychotic agent such as haloperidol (Haldol) or chlorpromazine (Thorazine)
   B. Lithium carbonate
   C. Chlordiazepoxide (Librium)
   D. None of the above
4. Lithium carbonate can:

A. Abort a manic attack
B. Decrease craving for alcohol and block an alcohol high
C. Prevent further manic attacks
D. Prevent further depressive attacks
E. Be ineffective
F. All of the above

Discussion

Symptoms of mania include irritability, paranoia, euphoria, logorrhea, manipulativeness, flight of ideas, grandiosity, hypersexuality, and insomnia. Manic patients tend to get themselves into trouble by acting out their impulses. The differential diagnosis between mania and acute paranoid schizophrenia is often difficult and may need to be made on the basis of historical factors and retrospectively. Severe mania is best initially managed in an inpatient setting by acutely treating the patient with an antipsychotic agent. Lithium carbonate should be started at the same time, but often will not exert its antimanic effects for 1 to 2 weeks. In cases of mild mania, lithium carbonate alone may be used. Lithium carbonate is a very effective treatment for acute mania, given enough time, and is useful in preventing future manic and depressive attacks. It is not effective in 100% of cases. Lithium carbonate has been reported useful in the treatment of alcoholism in which it appears to block the alcohol high and decrease the craving of alcohol.

Answers

1. (D)
2. (A)
3. (B)
4. (F)

References

1. Taylor, M. A. and Abrams, R.: Prediction of treatment response in mania. *Archives of General Psychiatry*, 38: 800–805, 1981.

2. Davis, J. M., Janowsky, D. S., and El-Yousef, M. K.: The use of lithium in clinical psychiatry. *Psychiatric Annals*, 3(2): 78–99, 1973.
3. Waters, B. G. and LaPierre, Y. D.: Therapeutic use of the tricyclic-induced switch in bipolar manic–depression. *American Journal of Psychiatry*, 139(2): 245–246, 1982.

CASE 28: PROPHYLACTIC LITHIUM CARBONATE TREATMENT

A 42-year-old woman, hospitalized in the nursing home portion of a state hospital, gives a 15-year history of frequent bipolar manic–depressive attacks. She has been treated with ECT, barbiturates, phenothiazines, and insulin-coma therapy. A decision is made to start lithium carbonate treatment. She is currently euthymic (neither depressed nor manic).

1. The lithium carbonate serum level that should be attained for prophylaxis in a euthymic patient is in the range of:
   A. 0.2 to 0.6 mEq/liter
   B. 0.7 to 1.0 mEq/liter
   C. 1.1 to 1.4 mEq/liter
   D. 1.5 to 1.8 mEq/liter
2. A dose of 900 to 1800 mg per day of lithium carbonate will probably be sufficient to produce an adequate serum level in this patient. The following is also true:
   A. If the patient were depressed, more drug would be necessary to obtain a given serum level
   B. If the patient were manic, more lithium carbonate would be necessary to obtain a given serum level
   C. If the patient were receiving a chlorothiazide diuretic, more lithium carbonate would be needed to obtain a given serum level
   D. If the patient were on a restricted-sodium diet, more lithium carbonate would be needed to obtain a given serum level
3. If the patient were acutely manic, the serum lithium carbonate level would most desirably be in the range of:
   A. 0.3 to 0.6 mEq/liter
   B. 0.7 to 1.0 mEq/liter

C. 1.1 to 1.4 mEq/liter
D. 1.5 to 1.8 mEq/liter

4. If the patient had obtained an adequate serum lithium carbonate level, and suddenly became depressed or euthymic, the serum lithium level would:
   A. Increase
   B. Decrease
   C. Stay the same
   D. All are likely with equal frequency
5. In the elderly patient, therapeutic and side effects of lithium carbonate are most likely to occur at:
   A. Lower doses and serum levels than in younger patients
   B. Higher doses and serum levels than in younger patients
   C. The same doses and serum levels than in younger patients

Discussion

The doses and serum levels of lithium that should be attained in treating a patient with bipolar illness vary with the patient's clinical status. Acutely, manic patients require higher serum levels of lithium (1.1 to 1.5 mEq/liter) to attain effects. Maintenance lithium serum levels should be in the range of 0.7 to 1.0 mEq/liter. Individuals vary considerably and may require more or less than the above amounts. Patients who are manic have an expanded "lithium space" and require more lithium carbonate to attain a given serum level. The converse is true when a patient is depressed. Sodium depletion from dietary restrictions and from chlorothiazide diuretics causes a compensatory retention of lithium carbonate, which can increase serum lithium levels and cause toxicity. Thus, patients on lithium carbonate who begin diets or diuretics should be carefully monitored. Lithium carbonate is more effective and more toxic in the elderly at lower doses than in younger patients, and should be used with caution. Lithium carbonate has a relatively low therapeutic/toxic ratio, and thus should be carefully monitored. Initially, the serum lithium level should be obtained every 2 to 3 days or more frequently. When a stable serum level is obtained, samples for serum lithium assay may be drawn every two weeks and later, once each month.

Answers

1. (B)
2. (B)
3. (C)
4. (A)
5. (A)

References

1. Shader, R. I.: *Manual of Psychiatric Therapeutics.* Little, Brown and Co., Boston, 1976.
2. Davis, J. M., Janowsky, D. S., and El-Yousef, M. K.: The use of lithium in clinical psychiatry. *Psychiatric Annals*, 3(2): 78–99, 1973.

CASE 29: ELECTROCONVULSIVE THERAPY IN AN ELDERLY PATIENT

The patient is a 64-year-old man with no psychiatric history prior to 3 weeks ago. Four weeks before your seeing him he suffered a myocardial infarction. Before that, he was a hard-working, moderately successful small-business proprietor. He recovered well from his acute myocardial infarction and was transferred out of the coronary intensive care unit. However, his family and the medical staff noted that he was withdrawn, uncommunicative, and appeared sad. Over the 3 subsequent weeks, his depression worsened, he refused to eat or ambulate, and asked to die. His medical condition began to deteriorate but his cardiac dysfunction was not severe enough to explain the picture. At this point you are called in as a consultant. Your mental-staus examination and history reveal a severely depressed man without signs of organic brain syndrome.

1. Which of the following medications or medical conditions have been shown to produce a picture like this?
   A. Cortisone
   B. Hyperparathyroidism
   C. Hypothyroidism
   D. Methyldopa (Aldomet)
   E. All of the above

Discussion

There are a large number of medical disorders that present with affective symptomatology, among which is hypothyroidism. In addition, a number of medications have been reported to be associated with depressive syndromes, including cortisone and antihypertensive medications, especially reserpine, alpha-methyldopa, and clonidine. Patients who receive reserpine are prone to present with severe depressive syndromes, which have endogenous features and may continue after the reserpine is stopped. This syndrome may require antidepressants or electroconvulsive therapy (ECT) for its alleviation. Cortisone and adrenocorticotropic hormone (ACTH) are most frequently associated with mood changes in the direction of cheerfulness and euphoria, but depression is also seen.

2. You consider using ECT. Which of the following statements affecting your choice of treatments is true?
   A. One absolute contraindication to ECT is increased intracranial pressure
   B. You are reluctant to use drug modified ECT because a full-blown convulsion will give your patient a better chance for recovery from his depression than a modified seizure
   C. ECT has been reported to be relatively safe in patients recuperating from myocardial infarction
   D. ECT really offers no advantages over tricyclic antidepressants

Discussion

Electroconvulsive therapy is a relatively safe procedure in selected patients. The only absolute contraindication to its use is an increase in intracranial pressure, and treatments have been successfully given to women in their first trimesters of pregnancy, and in patients recuperating from open-heart surgery or myocardial infarctions. Statistics show that complications occur in only one of every 2,600 treatments, and fatalities in one out of every 28,000.

3. Factors which have been reported to be associated with a relatively better response to ECT for the treatment of depression include:
   A. Slow onset of symptoms

B. Delirium
C. Visual hallucinations
D. Psychomotor retardation

Discussion

While some patients respond better to ECT than drugs, these cases are difficult to predict in advance. Attempts to predict ECT responsiveness on the basis of biologic tests or psychological examinations rest mainly with the patient's age, personality, or symptoms. The value of many of these tests, however, cannot be confirmed. One factor which seems to be prevalent in most studies of the predictiveness of the efficacy of ECT is a relatively slow onset of symptoms.

4. You decide to use ECT. Your orders for using the treatment are likely to include:
   A. Succinyl choline about 0.5 mg/kg
   B. A current of 240 V for the average patient
   C. Daily treatments
   D. Atropine 0.6 mg i.m. at the time of treatment

Discussion

In addition to a short-acting barbiturate and succinyl choline, atropine 0.6 mg is given subcutaneously or intramuscularly 30 to 60 minutes before treatment, both to prevent cardiac arrhythmias produced by vagal stimulation and to diminish the secretion (and thus the potential aspiration) of saliva. Treatments can then be given either unilaterally using the nondominant temporal region or bilaterally, where the electrodes are placed on the anterior portion of both temples. There is some indication that the duration and intensity of the current applied correlates with the severity of postconvulsive memory disturbances; in most instances the desired response can be achieved by delivery of 80 to 140 V of alternating current for 0.1 to 0.8 seconds. The amount of current that passes through the brain is estimated to be between 200 to 1,600 mA. Electroconvulsive therapy is usually given two or three times weekly and is best monitored with newer equipment that measures activity to insure occurrence of brain seizures.

5. Correct statements about the type of side effects your patient is likely to have include:
   A. There is a 50% chance of finding small punctate scars in the temporal cortex if more than 20 treatments are given
   B. Fractures, particularly at the sacral spine, are not uncommon even in drug modified ECT
   C. The risk of death is about 1%
   D. There may be an anterograde amnesia that remits gradually

Discussion

While there is a paucity of long-term studies to prove the safety of ECT, efforts to find permanent morphologic brain changes have been inconclusive. The most frequent complications in ECT prior to the introduction of succinylcholine were fractures, especially of the dorsal spine between the fourth and eighth vertebrae, but these have almost totally disappeared with the use of succinylcholine. Among the most disturbing side effects occurring with ECT is confusion. The more treatments the patient receives, the longer and more severe the confusional episodes become. Also, the more treatments, the further back the patient's memory disturbance extends and the more globally disoriented the patient becomes. The memory difficulty seems to be an anterograde amnesia, which remits gradually. The most gross symptoms of disorientation usually recede within a few weeks of the final treatment, but there may be total lack of memory for events occurring around the time of the treatment itself.

6. Correct statements about the effectiveness of ECT include:
   A. It usually effectively controls the thought disorder in chronic schizophrenics
   B. It is probably more rapidly effective than tricyclic antidepressants in treating depression
   C. It is more effective in curing depression if phenothiazines are given concomitantly
   D. It is usually effective in alleviating acute catatonia

Discussion

The relative effectiveness of ECT and tricyclic antidepressants is difficult to evaluate, because blind control studies are difficult to perform. However, many authors find that ECT works more rapidly and may be more effective than tricyclics. The only disorders for which ECT has been demonstrated to be repeatedly effective are affective disorders. One other disorder for which ECT is indicated is the acute catatonic state, where the patient's behavior is dangerous to himself or to those around him. It is difficult to determine whether this acute catatonic state is a schizophrenic reaction or a severe and precipitous onset of psychomotor retardation due to depression. Electroconvulsive therapy has no proven efficacy in the control of thought disorder in chronic schizophrenics, nor is there any indication that the effectiveness of the treatments are improved with the concomitant administration of major tranquilizers.

7. Factors that make ECT the treatment of choice in depression include:
   A. A patient in the first trimester of pregnancy
   B. A severe, rapidly progressing, incapacitating course of depression
   C. A desire to get the patient out of the hospital as quickly as possible
   D. A patient who has had prior episodes of depression that did not respond to tricyclics or monoamine oxidase inhibitors (MAOIs).

Discussion

There are a number of instances in which ECT is to be preferred over antidepressants in the treatment of a patient with an affective disorder. These include a patient in the first trimester of pregnancy, since it is probably true that ECT therapy is of less danger to the fetus than is the continued use of tricyclic antidepressants. In addition, a severely progressing, incapacitating course of illness may indicate that the patient cannot wait the necessary 2 to 4 weeks for a clinical response, making ECT the probable treatment of choice. Also, because ECT works more rapidly, a patient whose hospitalization must be as short as possible should probably have this therapy in preference to antidepressants. A final indication is a patient whose prior episode of depression did not respond to tricyclics but did respond to ECT.

Answers

1. (E)
2. (A and C)
3. (A and D)
4. (A and D)
5. (D)
6. (B and D)
7. (A, B, C, and D)

References

1. Hardman, J. B. and Morse, R. M.: Early electroconvulsive treatment of a patient who had artificial aortic and mitral valves. *American Journal of Psychiatry*, 128: 895–897, 1972.
2. Fink, M.: *Convulsive Therapy: Theory and Practice*. Raven Press, New York, 1979.
3. A.P.A. Task Force Fourteen: *Electroconvulsive Therapy, 1978*. American Psychiatric Association, Washington, D.C., 1978.
4. Klerman, G. L.: Depression in the medically ill patient. *Psychiatric Clinics of North America*, 4(2): 301–317, 1981.

CASE 30: TREATMENT OF PREMENSTRUAL TENSION

A 29-year-old woman who is the mother of three children becomes intensely irritable, tense, dysphoric, and mildly suicidal each month for about 1 week before and 3 days after onset of her menses. During one of these episodes, she argues with her husband and he leaves her to visit a woman friend. She promptly overdoses on her sleeping pills.

1. It is likely that a major biologic cause of this patient's affective symptoms is:
   A. Hypothyroidism
   B. Premenstrual tension
   C. Hyperventilation
   D. Hyperparathyroidism
2. Premenstrual tension, as a variable in causing suicidal behavior in women, is:

A. Often important
B. Relatively unimportant

3. Although no treatment has proven entirely satisfactory, the following treatment(s) may be useful in relieving the psychiatric symptoms of premenstrual tension:
A. Maintenance lithium carbonate
B. Low-dosage progestogen–estrogen oral contraceptives
C. Thiazide diuretics
D. Tricyclic antidepressants

Discussion

Premenstrual–menstrual affective disturbances are a very common phenomenon, occurring in up to 80% of women. During the premenstruum, suicidal behavior, psychotic episodes, bouts of alcoholism, crimes of violence, and most other psychopathogenic states occur at one and a half to two times their frequency in the rest of the menstrual cycle. Often, such behavior is unrecognized as linked to the menstrual cycle. Although no treatment has proven entirely satisfactory, there is some evidence that "premenstrual tension" is treatable with lithium carbonate maintenance therapy, low-dosage progestogen oral contraceptives, and maintenance tricyclic antidepressants. Thiazide diuretics have been used extensively to treat premenstrual tension, but these appear only to affect symptoms of water retention, and not the psychologic symptoms. A possible exception to this is the efficacy of spironolactone, as demonstrated in one controlled study.

Answers

1. (B)
2. (A)
3. (A, B, and D)

References

1. Dalton, K.: *The Premenstrual Syndrome*. William Heineman Medical Books, London, 1964.

2. Dalton, K.: Influence of menstruation on health and disease. *Proceedings of the Royal Society of London: Series B: Biological Sciences*, 57: 262–264, 1964.
3. Janowsky, D., Gorney, R., and Kelley, B.: The curse: I. Vicissitudes and variations of the female fertility cycle. *Psychosomatics*, 7: 242–246, 1966.
4. Rausch, J. L., Janowsky, D. S., Risch, S. C., Judd, L. L., and Huey, L. Y.: Hormonal and neurotransmitter hypotheses of premenstrual tension. *Psychopharmacology Bulletin*, 18(4): 25–34, 1982.

CASE 31: TREATMENT OF DEPRESSION IN AN ELDERLY WOMAN

The patient is a 72-year-old woman who is brought for psychiatric evaluation by her daughter, with whom she has been living for the past 2 years. The daughter reports that the woman was in good health and functioning well until approximately 4 months before the evaluation. At that time the patient slowly changed from being a rather outgoing, happy person to becoming someone who generally kept to herself and showed little interest in her usual activities. Over the past 4 months the patient has lost weight, has been noted to be irritable, has stopped participating in family activities, and at times, has been noted to be slow to understand concepts and to show a mild fluctuating confusion. The patient recently had a thorough physical and laboratory examination which was normal. A mental-status examination reveals a thin, nervous, sad-appearing woman, looking slightly older than her stated age. Her thoughts and responses seem to be quite slow. She shows no signs of hallucinations or delusions, and generally relates with a sad affect. She sees the future as hopeless, and shows mild impairment in her ability to think problems through and in her mathematical abilities.

1. The differential diagnosis of this patient includes:
   A. Atherosclerotic dementia
   B. Depression secondary to medical illness
   C. Senile dementia
   D. Major depressive disorder
   E. All of the above

Discussion

Any of the diagnoses listed above could present with an affective overlay to a confusional state, or the patient may appear confused secondarily to a primary affective disorder.

2. A working diagnosis of major depressive disorder is made. Correct statements about the treatment of this disorder in the elderly include:
   A. Monoamine oxidase inhibitors (MAOIs) are probably less indicated than tricyclic antidepressants, due to their side effects
   B. Patients with this disorder frequently present with confusion
   C. Patients with this disorder can present with apathy
   D. The majority of such patients will recover
   E. All of the above

Discussion

In the elderly, the clinical picture of depression varies considerably. However, the core group of signs and symptoms is similar in elderly and younger patients. The drug treatment of elderly patients is similar to the treatment of younger patients, and follows the same generalizations (e.g., MAOIs are probably less indicated than tricyclic antidepressants, due to their side effects, as an initial treatment, although they may actually be more efficacious). Elderly patients with affective disorders are more likely than younger patients to present with either confusion or apathy. Just as with their younger counterparts, it is probable that most elderly patients with depression will recover.

3. A decision is made to use electroconvulsive therapy (ECT) in this patient. Correct statements about this treatment in the elderly include:
   A. The average patient should be given two to three treatments a week
   B. Electroconvulsive therapy is not as effective as tricyclic antidepressants or monoamine oxidase inhibitors in this age group
   C. This treatment is remarkably safe in this age group, with few contraindications
   D. A and C

Discussion

Before using ECT in elderly patients, a thorough evaluation of their overall physical status is required, with particular attention given to the cardiovascular system. Age alone is not a contraindication to ECT. As with younger patients, ECT is probably the most effective mode of treatment for depression. A patient should be given two to three treatments a week until six to eight or more treatments have been given.

4. If the patient were to be treated with antidepressants, correct statements about treatment would include:
   A. The tricyclic antidepressants do not work for depression associated with Parkinson's disease
   B. It is not uncommon for some patients in this age group to require 250 mg imipramine (Tofranil) per day
   C. With this age group, one should begin the antidepressant drugs at the same dose as one would with younger patients
   D. The side effect of drowsiness usually disappears within several days to a week after the beginning of treatment with tricyclic antidepressants

Discussion

The same general guidelines apply to the use of antidepressant medications in the elderly as are applicable in younger patients. However, extra care must be taken regarding hypotensive problems, glaucoma, and urinary retention. While initial antidepressant-drug doses should always be relatively low (with imipramine begun at 30 to 100 mg per day or less, in divided doses), these doses may have to be slowly increased over a period of 3 to 5 days, to a dose of 125 to 150 mg per day. Doses of 250 mg may have to be used if the patient can tolerate the side effects. Thus, in summary, one should always begin elderly patients at lower doses of tricyclic antidepressants, because of possibly increased side effects. The final doses used may sometimes be the same or less than those required by younger patients.

5. Correct statements about the general treatment of an episode of affective illness in the elderly include:

A. The chances of suicide are higher in this age group than in younger age groups
B. With antidepressants, blurred vision may persist when the treatment is continued
C. One may see a decrease in nocturia with antidepressant-drug treatment
D. All of the above

Discussion

Other differences between elderly and younger patients with affective disorders include: (1) elderly patients probably have a higher rate of suicide; (2) some side effects, such as blurred vision, may persist longer in elderly patients. Another side effect of these drugs may be a decrease in nocturia, a property that allows these drugs to be used to treat enuresis.

Answers

1. (E)
2. (E)
3. (D)
4. (B and D)
5. (D)

References

1. Pfeiffer, E. and Busse, E. W.: Mental disorders in later life: Affective disorders. In: *Mental Illness in Later Life* (eds.: E. W. Busse and E. Pfeiffer). American Psychiatric Association, Washington, D.C., 1973.
2. Georgotas, A., Friedman, E., McCarthy, M., *et al.*: Resistant geriatric depressions and therapeutic response to monoamine oxidase inhibitors. *Biological Psychiatry*, 18: 195–205, 1983.
3. Ashford, J. W. and Ford, C. V.: Use of MAO inhibitors in elderly patients. *American Journal of Psychiatry*, 136: 1466–1467, 1979.
4. Caine, E.: Pseudodementia. *Archives of General Psychiatry*, 38: 1359, 1981.
5. Pitts, W. M., Fann, W. E., Sajadi, C., and Snyder, S.: Alprazolam in older inpatients. *Journal of Clinical Psychiatry*, 44: 213–215, 1983.

6. Veith, R. C.: Depression in the elderly: Pharmalogic considerations in treatment. *Journal of the American Geriatric Society*, 30: 581–596, 1982.
7. Gerner, R., Estabrook, W., Steuer, J., and Jarvik, L.: Treatment of geriatric depression with trazodone, imipramine and placebo: A double-blind study. *Journal of Clinical Psychiatry*, 41: 216–220, 1980.
8. McAllister, T. W.: Severe pseudodepression pseudodementia with and without dementia. *American Journal of Psychiatry*, 138: 626, 1982.

CASE 32: UTILIZATION OF ANTIDEPRESSANTS IN THE ELDERLY

You are called as a consultant in the case of a 66-year-old electrical engineer. The man was well until 6 months earlier when he noted having decreased energy, some depression, and a lowered level of stamina. His internist was beginning a medical workup but wanted an evaluation of the patient's depression.

1. Possible diagnoses include:
   A. Major depression
   B. Cancer of the head of the pancreas
   C. An intracranial neoplasm
   D. Addison's disease

Discussion

In establishing the diagnosis of an affective disorder, one must clearly keep in mind the difference between affective symptomatology and the diagnosis of major depression. There are a number of disorders which can present with sadness as the primary symptomatology, or even with major affective disorder, including a number of physiologic disorders, such as cancer of the head of the pancreas, brain tumors including meningiomas, and many hormonal imbalances, such as Sheehan's disease and Addison's disease.

2. The tests were all normal except for a cholesterol of 335 mg%, a T4 of 2.0 mEq/liter, with a T3 of 25% retention (both low levels). The internist completed a thyroid workup and began therapy, but wants

to know the general risks involved in using tricyclic-antidepressant medications. Your advice includes:

A. A risk of the development of a withdrawal syndrome consisting of akathisia, nausea, headache, or malaise if the drugs are stopped abruptly exists
B. A less than 5% rate of severe major adverse psychologic reactions (including psychosis and agitation) exists
C. A risk of precipitating a mania, especially in bipolar patients exists
D. All of the above

Discussion

The antidepressants are drugs that should only be given when indicated, but when indicated, the rate of side effects associated with their use is low enough to generally justify their use. The overall adverse reaction rate to these drugs is about 15%, as established by the Boston Collaborative Drug Surveillance Program. The major adverse reactions, such as psychosis, hallucinations, disorientation, and agitation occurred in less than 5% of the 260 patients studied. Data from 80 patients with preexisting cardiovascular disease showed no evidence of an increased mortality rate. In administering tricyclic antidepressants to patients with bipolar affective illness, one runs an additional risk. It is possible that the tricyclic antidepressants may precipitate mania, and this must be watched for carefully. There is also some indication that relatively long administration of these drugs may be followed by a cholinergic rebound withdrawal syndrome which includes malaise, nausea, and headache when the drugs are abruptly terminated. If this syndrome develops, it can be simply treated by reinstating the tricyclic antidepressant, and weaning the patient from the drug over a 1- to 2-week period.

3. The patient is 66 years old. If you had used antidepressants, what special precautions might you have to take with this age group?
   A. The overall clinical experience with tricyclics antidepressants in elderly patients shows them of great danger to this population
   B. Orthostatic hypotension is not an increased danger in the elderly population
   C. Monoamine oxidase inhibitors (MAOIs) have been shown in some controlled studies to be more effective than tricyclics in elderly patients

D. It is reasonable to give levels of 100 mg imipramine within 4 or 5 days of starting treatment in geriatric patients, if the patient is monitored for side effects

Discussion

The majority of elderly patients with depressive illness can be treated on the same basis as younger patients. Since physical illness occurs frequently in the older age group, however, a detailed physical examination should be made in every case. Antidepressant drugs are the treatment of choice for the majority of cases of depression in the elderly, with imipramine-type drugs starting at 25 mg, t.i.d. or less and raised in 4 or 5 days to 100 to 150 mg daily, with careful observation for side effects. However, many elderly patients will require considerably lower doses, and develop side effects at higher doses. In treating elderly patients, special care must be taken for their vulnerability to urinary retention, glaucoma, and orthostatic hypotension.

4. Thyroid medications are at times used for treating depressed patients. Correct statements about their use include:
   A. Both T3 and thyroid stimulating hormone (TSH) always show mild antidepressant actions when given alone
   B. A major use of T3 and T4 is to accelerate the response to antidepressants
   C. The probable action of T3 when used with imipramine is via a negative feedback mechanism on the hypothalamic–pituitary axis
   D. T3 daily is occasionally effective if used with imipramine, especially in young women

Discussion

In general it can be said that T3 (given in doses of 25 μg daily), and T4 have been shown to accelerate the response to imipramine-type drugs, especially in women. However, none of these drugs has been shown to be consistently effective on their own in the treatment of affective disorders in euthyroid patients. The mechanism for this enhancement of effects of tricyclic antidepressants is unknown and has been demonstrated to occur irrespective of the hypothalamic–pituitary axis.

Answers

1. (A, B, C, and D)
2. (D)
3. (C and D)
4. (B and D)

References

1. Coppen, A., Peet, S., Montgomery, S., *et al.*: Thyrotropin-releasing hormone in the treatment of depression. *Lancet*, 2: 433–435, 1974.
2. Prange, A. J., Wilson, E. C., Knox, A., *et al.*: Enhancement of imipramine by thyroid stimulating hormone: Clinical and theoretical implications. *American Journal of Psychiatry*, 127: 191–199, 1970.
3. Greenblatt, D. J., Sellers, E. M., and Shader, R. I.: Drug disposition in old age. *New England Journal of Medicine*, 306: 1081–1088, 1982.
4. Janowsky, D. S.: Management of depression in the elderly. *Journal of Family Practice Recertification*, 4(1) (Supplement): 37–48, 1982.
5. Thompson, T. L., Moran, M. G., and Nies, A. S.: Psychotropic drug use in the elderly: II. *New England Journal of Medicine*, 308: 194–199, 1983.
6. Foster, J. R., Gershell, W. J., and Coloxarb, A. I.: Lithium treatment in the elderly: I. Clinical usage. *Journal of Gerontology*, 32: 299–302, 1977.
7. Nies, A., Robinson, D. S., Friedman, M. J., *et al.*: Relationship between age and tricyclic antidepressant plasma levels. *American Journal of Psychiatry*, 134: 790–793, 1977.
8. Veith, R. C., Raskind, M. A., Caldwell, J., *et al.*: Cardiovascular effects of tricyclic antidepressants in depressed patients with chronic heart disease. *New England Journal of Medicine*, 306: 954–959, 1982.
9. Georgotas, A., Friedman, E., McCarthy, M., *et al.*: Resistant geriatric depressions and therapeutic response to monoamine oxidase inhibitors. *Biological Psychiatry*, 18: 195–205, 1983.
10. Ashford, J. W. and Ford, C. V.: Use of MAO inhibitors in elderly patients. *American Journal of Psychiatry*, 136: 1466–1467, 1979.
11. Katon, W. and Raskind, M.: Treatment of depression in the medically ill elderly with methylphenidate. *American Journal of Psychiatry*, 137: 963–965, 1980.
12. Kaufman, M. W., Murray, G. B., and Cassem, N. H.: Use of psychostimulants in medically ill depressed patients. *Psychosomatics*, 23: 817–819, 1982.
13. Clark, A. G. and Mankikar, G. D.: D-Amphetamine in elderly patients; refractory to rehabilitation procedures. *Journal of the American Geriatric Society*, 27: 174–177, 1979.

14. Sabelli, H. C., Fawcett, J., Javaid, J. I., and Bagri, S.: The methylphenidate test for differentiating desipramine-responsive from nortriptyline-responsive depression. *American Journal of Psychiatry*, 140: 212–214, 1983.
15. Goodwin, F. K., Prange, A. J., Post, R. M., Muscettola, G., Lipton, M. A.: Potentiation of antidepressant effects by L-triiodothyronine in tricyclic non-responders. *American Journal of Psychiatry*, 139: 34–38, 1982.
16. Prange, A. J., Wilson, C., Rabon, A. M., and Lipton, M. A.: Enhancement of imipramine antidepressant activity by thyroid hormone. *American Journal of Psychiatry*, 126: 457, 1969.

CASE 33: TREATMENT OF MANIA IN THE ELDERLY

A 67-year-old man is brought to the emergency room of the hospital. His wife relates that he had been functioning well until approximately 3 days prior to his admission. At that time he rather rapidly became nervous, with increased amounts of energy, decreased sleeping time, and increasing levels of confusion. He has had grandiose ideas, with thoughts of entering expensive business ventures, and feels that he has been given special powers by God to carry out a number of important missions. A mental-status examination shows the patient to be alert and speaking at a very rapid rate. He is quite difficult to interrupt, and has very loose associations and a generally euphoric affect. At times the patient is irritable.

1. Correct statements about this illness include:
   A. Mania rarely, if ever, occurs in old age
   B. The picture could be explained by amphetamine abuse
   C. This is a fairly typical history for the onset of process schizophrenia in old age
   D. One would expect a past history of psychiatric illness in this individual, but it does not have to exist

Discussion

Bipolar affective disorder is not limited to young patients. The onset of first manias has been reported throughout life, including the eighth and ninth decades. As is true with any of the psychiatric disorders, one should rule out the possibility of alcohol or drug abuse.

2. The immediate drug treatment of this patient may include:
   A. Thioridazine (Mellaril) 100 mg, q.i.d., increased rapidly to a dose of 1,200 to 1,300 mg per day as needed
   B. Haloperidol (Haldol) 10 to 20 mg per day or less
   C. If the patient were exquisitely sensitive to antipsychotic medications, one could consider using promethazine (Phenergan) 12.5 mg two to four times a day as an antimanic agent
   D. Major tranquilizers have been proven to be better than placebo in manic episodes

Discussion

The major tranquilizers are of use in elderly patients who demonstrate a manic picture. Small amounts of chlorpromazine or thioridazine can be used, beginning with 10 mg of either drug given q.i.d., which can be increased fairly rapidly to 200 mg per day or more. However, one must be especially careful to increase the dosage slowly in patients with marginal cerebral competence. The prophylactic use of antiparkinsonian medications along with phenothlazines is controversial. Anticholinergic drugs can complicate matters because of their agitating effects and their tendency to promote confusion. Major tranquilizers have been shown to help control the agitation and paranoid ideation that can occur in aged manic patients.

3. You decide that the diagnosis of a bipolar disorder, manic phase, is correct, and following the initiation of acute antipsychotic drug treatment you begin lithium therapy. Correct statements about the use of lithium in this age group include:
   A. The blood levels should be kept below 0.5 mEq/liter
   B. Moderate renal failure is an absolute contraindication to the use of lithium in older patients
   C. One must never combine lithium with major tranquilizers in older patients

D. There is no indication that lithium is any less effective in older than younger patients

Discussion

Lithium carbonate can be very effective in the treatment of mania in elderly patients. The same general guidelines used for lithium treatment in younger patients should be followed in the elderly. However, lower lithium levels often suffice in the elderly (i.e., 0.8 to 1.0 mEq/liter). Thus, lithium should be given initially at low dosages and increased slowly in the elderly. It can be used conjointly with antipsychotic drugs and antidepressants. The toxic effects of lithium in this age group, which may occur at lower serum levels, are similar to those in younger patients, and mild toxic reactions can be treated by discontinuing the lithium, urging the taking of fluids, and using supplemental sodium chloride p.o. Special caution is required with lithium in the presence of cardiac or renal disease.

4. Correct statements about the relative effectiveness of medications in the treatment of bipolar affective disease, manic phase in old age groups include:
   A. Haloperidol (Haldol) is superior to thioridazine (Mellaril)
   B. Chlorpromazine (Thorazine) is superior to haloperidol
   C. Trifluoperazine (Stelazine) is superior to haloperidol
   D. Fluphenazine (Prolixin) is generally equal in efficacy to perphenazine (Trilafon)

Discussion

There is little indication that any of the major tranquilizers are better than any of the others in elderly persons in the manic phase of a bipolar disorder, and the same general rule holds true for the tricyclic antidepressants. The specific medication chosen is usually based on the physician's past experience, as well as the specific patient's history. The drug is usually chosen because its side effects will be better tolerated by a given patient than will those of another drug.

Answers

1. (B and D)
2. (B and D)
3. (D)
4. (D)

References

1. Winokur, G., Clayton, P. J., and Reich, T.: *Manic Depressive Illness*. C.V. Mosby Co., St. Louis, MO, 1969.
2. Spring, G. and Frankel, M.: New data on lithium and haloperidol incompatibility. *American Journal of Psychiatry*, 138: 818–821, 1982.
3. Prakash, R., Kelwala, S., and Ban, T. A.: Neurotoxicity with combined administration of lithium and a neuroleptic. *Comprehensive Psychiatry*, 23: 567–571, 1982.
4. Greenblatt, D. J., Sellers, E. M., and Shader, R. I.: Drug disposition in old age. *New England Journal of Medicine*, 306: 1081–1088, 1982.
5. Foster, J. R., Gershell, W. J., and Goloxarb, A. I.: Lithium treatment in the elderly: I. Clinical usage. *Journal of Gerontology*, 32: 299–302, 1977.
6. Tosteson, D. C.: Lithium and mania. *Scientific American*, 244: 164–174, 1981.

CASE 34: INTERACTION OF IMIPRAMINE AND GUANETHIDINE

An 88-year-old man with severe hypertension is being maintained on guanethidine (Ismelin) for treatment of his elevated blood pressure. He becomes depressed and is placed on 200 mg imipramine (Tofranil) at bedtime. Medical problems then develop.

1. It is likely that the patient's blood pressure will:
   A. Increase
   B. Decrease
   C. Stay the same
2. An increase in blood pressure will occur because:
   A. Imipramine is an adrenergic drug

   B. Imipramine blocks the uptake of guanethidine into the neuron, thus blocking it from exerting its effect
   C. Imipramine releases all the norepinephrine from the neuron
3. Other drugs that can cause an antagonism of guanethidine effects include:
   A. Chlorpromazine (Thorazine)
   B. Haloperidol (Haldol)
   C. Methylphenidate (Ritalin)
   D. All of the above
4. Drugs that may lower the blood pressure in the presence of a tricyclic antidepressant are:
   A. Reserpine
   B. Alpha-methyldopa
   C. Chlorothiazide diuretics
   D. All of the above
   E. None of the above

Discussion

Guanethidine is taken up into its neuronal site of action by the same amine uptake pump that takes up norepinephrine. Since tricyclic antidepressants block this pump, they also block guanethidine's effect on the neuron. Therefore, guanethidine's hypotensive effect is blocked by a tricyclic antidepressant, and a blood pressure that has been previously controlled will increase. Any drug that blocks the membrane uptake pump can potentially block guanethidine's effects. These include phenothiazines and other antipsychotic agents, amphetamine-like compounds, and cocaine. Antihypertensive medications which are not taken up by the norepinephrine membrane uptake pump, such as reserpine, alpha-methyldopa, and the diuretics can be used effectively in conjunction with tricyclic antidepressants.

Answers

1. (A)
2. (B)
3. (D)
4. (D)

References

1. Janowsky, D. S., El-Yousef, M. K., Davis, J. M., and Fann, W. E.: Antagonism of guanethidine by chlorpromazine. *American Journal of Psychiatry*, 130(7): 808–812, 1973.
2. Risch, S. C., Groom, G., and Janowsky, D. S.: The effects of psychotropic drugs on the cardiovascular system. *Journal of Clinical Psychiatry*, 43: 16–31, 1982.
3. Risch, S. C., Groom, G., and Janowsky, D. S.: Interfaces of psychopharmacology and cardiology: II. *Journal of Clinical Psychiatry*, 42: 47–59, 1981.
4. Gaultieri, C. and Powell, S.: Psychoactive drug interactions. *Journal of Clinical Psychiatry*, 39: 720–829, 1978.

CASE 35: COMBINATION MONOAMINE OXIDASE INHIBITOR–TRICYCLIC ANTIDEPRESSANT THERAPY

The patient is a 34-year-old female in good physical health, with an incapacitating major depressive disorder of 4 years' duration. She has been refractory to treatment, with a slight improvement only following electroconvulsive therapy (ECT), a slight and temporary improvement with adequate doses of amitriptyline (Elavil) on one occasion, and with tranylcypromine (Parnate) on another. When you first see her she is depressed and suicidal, but has not been on medications. You decide to try a combination of amitryptyline and tranylcypromine.

1. Correct statements about the uses and proposed mechanism of action for the two drugs include:
   A. It is thought that tranylcypromine works primarily intracellularly to stop the breakdown of monoamines
   B. Tranylcypromine can be given both orally and in an injectable form
   C. It is thought that amitriptyline works to decrease the neuronal reuptake of monamines, with the net result being that more transmitter accumulates in the synaptic cleft
   D. Tranylcypromine has consistently been shown to be equal in efficacy to amitriptyline in treating depression

E. Both tranylcypromine and amitriptyline may "down-regulate" central-nervous-system beta-receptors

Discussion

The two most accepted pharmacologic treatments for affective disorder are the tricyclic and related antidepressants and the monoamine oxidase inhibitors (MAOIs). The tricyclics are available in both oral and injectable forms, although oral forms are almost exclusively used. The drugs are well absorbed from the digestive tract and rapidly metabolized, with only 3% being excreted in unchanged form. The mechanism of action for the tricyclic drugs is not known with certainty, but it is felt that they probably act by decreasing the reuptake of monoamines by neurons, with a resulting increased concentration of these chemicals in the synaptic cleft, followed by a "down-regulation" or decrease in cortical beta-receptors and a coincident antidepressant efficacy.

The term "monoamine oxidase inhibitors" is applied to diverse substances with a common property of inhibiting enzymes designated as monoamine oxidases. These enzymes are responsible for the intracellular breakdown of monoamines, and the proposed mechanism of action of the MAOIs in the treatment of depression is that they increase the amount of transmitter substance within the cell itself. The first MAOI used for depression was iproniazid, a drug which subsequently proved to have such hepatotoxic effects that it was abandoned. A number of other drugs have come on the market, the most frequent in use today being phenelzine (Nardil), tranylcypromine, and pargyline (Eutonyl). The MAOIs are readily absorbed from the digestive tract, but are not available in injectable form. They also cause a "down-regulation" of cortical beta-receptors, with a time course coincident with their antidepressant efficacy. Most controlled studies indicate that the tricyclic antidepressants are slightly superior to the MAOIs in the treatment of affective disorders.

2. The side effects of tranylcypromine include:
   A. Anticholinergic symptoms of a dry mouth, blurred vision, constipation, and tachycardia
   B. The possibility of hypertension, even in the absence of foods with a high tyramine content, which would be expected to cause hypertension

C. Potentiation of amphetamines, some diuretics, and antihistamines
D. Central nervous system effects such as seizures
E. All of the above

Discussion

The side effects of the MAOI drugs are in some ways similar to those of the tricyclic antidepressants. These include the possibility of converting a depression to a mania in patients with bipolar disorders; autonomic side effects such as dizziness, orthostatic hypotension, urinary retention, constipation, dry mouth; and adverse interactions with drugs such as amphetamines, some diuretics, and antihistamines. Hypertension can be seen with these drugs, even in the absence of the intake of tyramine, but the usual hypertensive crisis follows the ingestion of foods that contain tyramine, such as aged cheese, broad beans, beer, yeast products, Chianti wine, pickled herring, chocolate, or chicken livers. The reaction involves a sharp elevation in blood pressure, usually associated with a severe throbbing headache, nausea, fever, vomiting, sweating, and nuchal rigidity. In some cases the patient may develop a subarachnoid hemorrhage with an occasional fatal outcome.

3. Correct statements about the side effects of combined tricyclic antidepressant–MAOI therapy include:
   A. Large-scale outpatient studies have shown that these drugs careful combined use does not result in excessive morbidity
   B. The reported cases of adverse reactions to such combined therapy show clinical pictures similar to those in MAOI or tricyclic overdosage alone
   C. Adverse effects of the combination of tricyclic antidepressants with MAOIs are probably more frequent if the MAOI is used first
   D. All of the above

Discussion

The combination of tricyclic antidepressants and MAOIs has been reported effective in the treatment of depression, but this treatment is often avoided because of concern about adverse reactions. A review of the case reports on which this concern is based reveals no convincing evidence that the antidepressant combination, taken in therapeutic doses, was responsible for the reactions reported. An informal review of 350 outpatients, a medical-record examination of 50 inpatients, and a drug trial with 10 current patients has shown no drug-related morbidity. The authors of the review concluded that the evidence did not indicate that the combined drug regimen was unsafe. The answer is not totally in, however; and a suggestion is made for more controlled clinical trials of combined MAOI–tricyclic antidepressant therapy to better evaluate its clinical effectiveness. The adverse interaction between the two classes of antidepressant drugs is not greatly different from the toxic reactions seen with either drug alone. While the therapeutic efficacy of the combination has not been established, the combined drugs can be considered one treatment for severe depression resistant to MAOIs tricyclic drugs alone. Of course, all patients should be instructed to avoid high-tyramine foods as well as amphetamines and over-the-counter cold medications. If serious side effects should occur, because of sympathetic discharge, alpha-adrenergic blocking agents such as phentolamine or neuroleptics such as chlorpromazine are efficacious.

4. Correct statements about the efficacy of combined tricyclic antidepressant–MAOI therapy include:
   A. The majority of controlled studies show that the combination of these drugs is faster acting and more effective than either drug alone
   B. Most patients will respond to doses of 50 mg amitriptyline and 10 mg tranylcypromine daily
   C. Most patients who do respond to the combination do so within several hours of addition of the second drug
   D. The combined treatment may be effective for those patients with depression resistant to other modes of therapy

Discussion

It must be emphasized that only a very few controlled studies have demonstrated the efficacy of the combined antidepressant–MAOI regimen, and some studies have yielded negative results. Those studies yielding positive results have indicated that the combination may work faster and work in refractory patients. However, the important controlled studies are only beginning to be done. The improvement after addition of the second drug is fairly rapid, usually occurring within a week.

5. Correct statements about uncontrolled studies of the treatment of endogenous depression include:
   A. Most treatments will not look effective in uncontrolled studies unless they are truly effective
   B. The placebo response rate to antidepressant medication is between 15 and 25% or more
   C. One reason uncontrolled studies are difficult to evaluate is because many depressive patients will improve with no treatment at all
   D. Good controlled experiments eliminate almost all bias

Discussion

Antidepressant drug efficacy must be evaluated through controlled studies. The spontaneous remission rate for affective disorders is high, and almost any maneuver or medication may look effective because a high percentage of patients get well on their own. It is only through careful, controlled evaluations that one can be sure that the medication is the actual cause of an observed improvement.

Answers

1. (A, C, and E)
2. (E)
3. (D)
4. (D)
5. (B and C)

References

1. Smith, A., Tranganza, E., and Harrison, G.: Studies on the effectiveness of antidepressant drugs. *Psychopharmacology*, 5: 1–21, 1969.
2. Schuckit, M. A., Robins, E., and Feighner, J.: Tricyclic antidepressants and

monoamine oxidase inhibitors. *Archives of General Psychiatry*, 24: 509–514, 1971.
3. Sethna, E. R.: A study of refractory cases of depressive illness and their response to combined antidepressant treatment. *British Journal of Psychiatry*, 124: 265–272, 1974.
4. Winston, F.: Combined antidepressant therapy. *British Journal of Psychiatry*, 118: 301–304, 1971.
5. Razani, J., White, K. L., White, J., *et al.*: The safety and efficacy of combined amitriptyline and tranylcypromine antidepressant treatment. *Archives of General Psychiatry*, 40: 657–662, 1983.
6. White, K. and Simpson, G.: Combined MAOI–tricyclic antidepressant treatment: A reevaluation. *Journal of Clinical Psychopharmacology*, 1: 264–282, 1981.
7. Paykel, E. S., Rowan, P. R., Parker, R. R., and Bhat, A. V.: Response to phenelzine and amitriptyline in subtypes of outpatient depression. *Archives of General Psychiatry*, 39: 1041–1049, 1982.
8. Linnoila, M., George, L., and Guthrie, S.: Interaction between antidepressants and perphenazine in psychiatric inaptients. *American Journal of Psychiatry*, 139: 1329–1331, 1982.
9. Lader, M.: Combined use of tricyclic antidepressants and monoamine oxidase inhibitors. *Journal of Clinical Psychiatry*, 44: 20–24, 1983.
10. Ravaris, C. L., Robinson, D. S., Ives, J. O., Nies, A., and Bartlett, D.: Phenelzine and amitriptyline in the treatment of depression: A comparison of present and past studies. *Archives of General Psychiatry*, 37: 1075–1080, 1980.
11. Palmer, R.: The safety and efficacy of combined amitriptyline and tranylcypromine antidepressant treatment. *Archives of General Psychiatry*, 40: 657–662, 1983.
12. Quitkin, F., Rifkin, A., and Klein, D. F.: Monoamine oxidase inhibitors. *Archives of General Psychiatry*, 26: 749–760, 1979.

CASE 36: ANTIDEPRESSANT TREATMENT IN A HEMODIALYSIS PATIENT

You are called on to consult in the case of a 23-year-old man who is in a renal-dialysis unit. The patient has symptoms of agitation and depression and is threatening to stop all treatments. After talking to the patient and his family, you arrive at the diagnosis of major depressive disorder and recommend treatment.

1. You consider using a tricyclic antidepressant. Correct statements about the use of these drugs in patients with renal failure are that:
   A. The route of excretion of these drugs is almost totally hepatic
   B. The normal half-life for these drugs is under 3 hours
   C. Even in severe renal failure the dose schedule of these drugs is essentially the same as in normal persons
   D. Drug doses should probably be given every 2 hours

Discussion

Patients with impaired renal function frequently require major adjustments in their dosage of common therapeutic agents to avoid adverse reactions. This becomes quite complex in the case of psychotropic drugs, since dialysis patients often require some form of sedation. An article by Bennett *et al.* in the *Journal of the American Medical Association* discussed various drugs, their route of excretion, their normal half-life, the maintenance doses that should be used in renal-failure and other patients, and their dialysability, as well as remarking about the toxic effects of these medications. The tricyclic antidepressants generally have a hepatic mode of excretion and a relatively long half-life, although it should be noted that the half-life of different tricyclic antidepressants may vary considerably. The usual dosage of these medications can be given to patients who are in renal failure, with dose administration every 8 hours. These drugs respond partially to peritoneal dialysis if toxic levels are reached.

2. Properties of the tricyclic antidepressants that must be carefully considered in renal-dialysis patients include:
   A. The possibility of urinary retention due to anticholinergic effects
   B. The possible decrease in the hypotensive effects of antihypertensive drugs
   C. The fact that little of these drugs is excreted intact
   D. The fact that these drugs are very hepatotoxic

Discussion

In administering tricyclic antidepressants to patients in renal failure, the anticholinergic properties of these drugs should be kept in mind, as well as their interactions with antihypertensive medications, which usually decreases the effectiveness of the latter drugs. Unlike monoamine oxidase inhibitors, the tricyclic antidepressants are not known for their excessive hepatotoxicity. There is a great individual variability in metabolism of the tricyclic antidepressants, which should be taken into consideration in evaluating any patient, whether on dialysis or not. There can be anywhere from a 10- to a 40-fold difference in blood levels with the same dosage of the same medication from one individual to another—a variability which may be genetically influenced. In addition, there is at least a two-fold difference between individuals in the percentage of drug that is bound to protein in the blood. The excretion of these drugs is dependent upon metabolism.

3. Because of the patient's agitation, you also consider adding an antipsychotic agent. Correct statements about these drugs are that:
   A. Their excretion is at least 50% renal
   B. Their normal half-life is 16 hours
   C. In the presence of moderate to severe renal failure, they should be given only once in 36 hours
   D. These drugs are refractory to dialysis

Discussion

The review article by Bennett *et al.* indicates that the phenothiazine drugs are almost totally excreted by a hepatic route. Their normal half-life is under 3 hours, and their rate of excretion is little affected by renal failure. This group of drugs generally is not dialysable.

4. The patient's physician asks about the use of minor tranquilizers. Correct statements about minor tranquilizers in renal-dialysis patients are:
   A. The excretion of the diazepam (Valium) is almost totally hepatic
   B. The half-life of diazepam is under 3 hours
   C. Diazepam can be given in the presence of moderate to severe renal failure
   D. Chlordiazepoxide (Librium) is more efficacious than diazepam in treating anxiety in renal-dialysis patients

Discussion

Most minor tranquilizers, especially diazepam, are excreted almost totally through a hepatic route and their half-life is somewhere between 22 and 190 hours. The excretion of these drugs is not greatly changed in the presence of renal failure—a statement especially true for diazepam. There is no major difference between specific minor tranquilizers in their efficacy in treating agitation in dialysis patients.

5. The possibility that the patient may have a bipolar affective disorder is raised. You consider using lithium. Correct statements about the use of lithium in renal-dialysis patients include:
   A. Excretion of the drug is almost totally renal
   B. The normal half-life of the drug is between 12 and 48 hours
   C. The drug should be avoided in the presence of moderate to severe renal failure
   D. Toxic doses of the drug can be treated with dialysis

Discussion

Lithium carbonate is almost totally excreted by a renal route, with a half-life between 24 and 48 hours. While this drug can be given to patients in mild renal failure approximately every 8 hours, it should be avoided in anyone in whom moderate to severe renal failure exists. If toxic levels are reached, however, lithium can be dialyzed either by hemodialysis or peritoneal dialysis.

6. The patient is also having some severe trouble sleeping. Correct statements about hypnotics in the treatment of patients with renal failure include:
   A. In cases of toxic doses of the barbiturates, hemodialysis is at least two times as effective as peritoneal dialysis
   B. Benzodiazepines (e.g., flurazepam [Dalmane]) are greatly preferable to barbiturates as hypnotics, whether or not they are used in patients with renal failures
   C. Glutethimide (Doriden) should never be given in the presence of severe renal failure
   D. The barbiturates are primarily excreted by the kidney

Discussion

The properties of the barbiturate and nonbarbiturate sedative hypnotics vary with the individual medication, but a number of generalizations can be made. In general, for the sedative hypnotics, hemodialysis is at least twice as effective as peritoneal dialysis. Also, most of these drugs are excreted primarily through the hepatic route. Glutethimide is a drug that must be avoided in moderate to severe renal failure—a statement not true of the barbiturate drugs. Benzodiazepines are the medications of choice as hypnotics, and most clinicians believe barbiturates and glutethimide should not be used as hypnotics.

Answers

1. (A and C)
2. (A, B, and C)
3. (D)
4. (A and C)
5. (A, B, C, and D)
6. (A, B, and C)

References

1. Bennett, W. M., Singer, I., and Coggins, C. J.: A guide to drug therapy in renal failure: *Journal of the American Medical Association*, 230: 1544–1553, 1974.
2. Baldessarini, R. J.: *Chemotherapy in Psychiatry*. Harvard University Press, Cambridge, MA, 1977.
3. Meyer, J. D., McAllister, K., and Goldberg, L. I.: Insidious and prolonged antagonism of guanethidine by amitriptyline. *Journal of the American Medical Association*, 213: 1487–1488, 1970.
4. Glassman, A. J.: The clinical pharmacology of imipramine. *Archives of General Psychiatry*, 28: 649–653, 1973.
5. Klerman, G. L.: Depression in the medically ill patient. *Psychiatric Clinics of North America*, 4(2): 301–317, 1981.

CASE 37: DIAGNOSIS AND TREATMENT OF MANIA IN AN ELDERLY WOMAN

Mrs. O. is a 71-year-old married woman with a history of two previous episodes of depression diagnosed as major affective disturbance, depressed. Her husband states that she has been without psychiatric treatment for the past 5 years. Three months previously, soon after their return from a European cruise to celebrate their 45th anniversary, the patient's husband noted a significant change in her behavior. He states that she initially became increasingly insomniac and hyperactive. On the day prior to his calling your office, she phoned the U.S. Embassy in Paris and made numerous long-distance calls complaining of various international American relationships. She was also planning to have a "reunion" for the entire ship at her home over the next week. Her demands accelerated when her husband refused to call the potential guests. She left the house for errands that accomplished little, and made frequent calls to her neighbors. An appointment is made with you at your office. Upon examination, Mrs. O.'s speech is pressured and tangential. Her appearance is disorganized. She speaks loudly and demands your total attention, frequently criticizing her husband for "thinking small" and refusing to agree to the "grand party." According to her husband, she now has a provocative manner, unlike that of her premorbid personality. She goes on to explain that she feels she has "special political" influence in several important countries. She feels you need to be more important if you are to be her doctor.

1. The probable diagnosis is:
   A. Schizophrenic disorder, paranoid type
   B. Major affective disturbance, bipolar, manic
   C. Organic delusional syndrome
   D. Brief reactive psychosis

Discussion

With a history of preexisting affective disorder, the most likely diagnosis is major affective disturbance, bipolar type, reflected by an episode of manic psychosis. Without a previously existing thought disorder and overt paranoid ideation, schizophrenic disorder is unlikely. Since the patient has undergone a rapid change in behavior over the previous week, and there is no evidence of specific cognitive dysfunction, diagnosing an organic delusional syndrome would be incorrect. Although a brief reactive psychosis might occur after a significant stress, such as a trip, the possibility of this occurring months after the patient's return, and in the presence of a preexisting affective disturbance, would make this diagnosis unlikely.

2. Correct statements about this patient's illness are that:
   A. Mania rarely occurs in later life
   B. The symptoms could be accounted for by amphetamine abuse
   C. The history is typical for the onset of schizophrenia in old age
   D. A past history of psychiatric illness is expected but not essential

Discussion

The first onset of major affective illness can occur at any age. The onset of first manic attacks have been reported throughout life, including the eighth and ninth decades. Drugs and alcohol can cause manic-like psychosis, and their role as causative agents of such an illness must not be ruled out.

3. Correct statements describing the immediate drug treatment of this patient include:
   A. Thioridazine, in small doses increased slowly as needed, is indicated
   B. Haloperidol, in low doses, decreased after improvement, is indicated
   C. Major tranquilizers have proven to be better than placebos in treating major affective disturbance of the bipolar type

Discussion

The major tranquilizers are of use in patients who demonstrate manic symptoms. Small amounts of chlorpromazine or thioridazine can be used, and the dose increased if the drug is clinically tolerated. However, one must be especially careful to increase the dosage slowly in patients with medical illness or signs of marginal cerebral competence. In general, the prophylactic use of antiparkinsonian medications is unnecessary, especially in the elderly. These anticholinergic drugs may complicate matters because of their agitating effects and tendency to promote paranoia and confusion. Antipsychotic drugs such as haloperidol, with less sedating effects, may be useful.

4. Lithium, as a treatment of choice, is contraindicated in patients older than 65 years of age:
   A. True
   B. False

Discussion

There are various approaches to this patient. The use of antipsychotic medications such as haloperidol or chlorpromazine for the acute manic phases of the patient's illness should be considered. Lithium is not contraindicated because of the patient's age. Equating age with illness is inaccurate, and various physiological parameters should be considered in treating the elderly, rather than stereotyping them. A direct correlation between chronology and biology does not exist in a given individual, and there are wide variations in individual physiological function with increasing age.

5. As a consequence of aging, the following physiological changes occur which directly affect the patient's capacity to tolerate and utilize drugs. Indicate ↑ for "increase" and ↓ for "decrease."
   A. Cardiac output
   B. Renal blood flow
   C. Hepatic enzyme activity
   D. Concentration of albumin relative to globulin
   E. Time necessary for absorption from the gastrointestinal tract

Discussion

The pharmacokinetics of drug utilization in the elderly are affected by various physiological parameters. Cardiac output decreases with age, as does renal blood flow, glomerular filtration, hepatic-enzyme activity, and the ratio of serum albumin to globulin. Absorption from the gastrointestinal tract diminishes with age, with an increased amount of time necessary for adequate absorption. The consequences of the above are a prolonged drug elimination and half-life, a reduction in total drug clearance, and an increased unbound drug concentration due to decreased binding.

6. The following factor is most critical to the effective utilization of lithium:
   A. Cardiac output
   B. Renal glomerular filtration
   C. Gastrointestinal absorption
   D. The albumin-to-globulin serum ratio

Discussion

As much as a 30% decrease in glomerular filtration and creatine clearance occurs with normal aging. In younger patients the half-life of lithium is 18 to 30 hours. In the elderly, it may be as long as 36 hours. Therefore, a 50% decrease in dosage may be necessary to compensate for reduced renal clearance in older patients.

Case Continued: In giving her medical history, Mrs. O. states that she has been taking hydrochlorothiazide 50 mg per day for hypertension. On admission her blood pressure is 150/90 mm Hg and her pulse is 80 and regular.

7. The most reasonable treatment strategy at this point would be to:
   A. Discontinue the hydrochlorothiazide
   B. Increase the hydrochlorothiazide
   C. Discontinue lithium therapy
   D. Consider using a higher dosage of lithium
   E. Consider using a lower dosage of lithium

Discussion

The combined use of most diuretics and lithium may reduce lithium clearance. Thiazide diuretics produce a distal diuresis of sodium leading to an increased reabsorption of lithium. This medication combination can be used, but only with appropriate caution. Adequate sodium intake should be maintained and proper monitoring of lithium levels must be done. The aldosterone antagonist spironolactone, a substance which acts on the distal renal tubules and leaves the proximal renal tubules unaffected, is unlikely to cause lithium retention. In view of this, some authors recommend spironolactone as the diurectic of choice for patients on lithium treatment.

8. An intitial starting dose of lithium per day in this patient could be:
   A. 150 to 300 mg p.o., b.i.d.
   B. 300 mg p.o., b.i.d.
   C. 600 mg p.o., t.i.d.

Discussion

In the elderly, the elimination half-life of lithium may be increased. A steady serum level may not occur for a week or more following initiation of therapy. Serum levels measured prior to obtaining a steady drug state should not be used as a guide to dosage. As a treatment strategy in the elderly, changes in the lithium dosage should occur only after the blood levels have been shown to have attained a steady state. General principles of treatment in the elderly suggest that slow changes in dosage are indicated.

Case Continued: Three weeks after you initiate treatment, the patient has shown a significant improvement in mood. Her personality has returned to its premorbid state, and her present serum lithium level is 1.0 mEq/liter.

9. Issues affecting lithium maintenance in the elderly are that:
   A. The elderly have a higher risk for lithium toxicity at therapeutic levels
   B. Some studies have suggested the elderly may have higher intracellular lithium concentrations
   C. Older patients may do well on lower maintenance levels (0.4 to 0.6 mEq/liter or less)

D. Lithium intoxication can occur at therapeutic levels in older patients
E. All of the above

Discussion

Lithium intoxication, especially with regard to neurological symptoms such as tremor, confusion, and dyskinesia, can occur at therapeutic levels in elderly patients. Targeting the lower spectrum of maintenance serum levels to prevent recurrence of a major affective disturbance would seem appropriate. Aging in some patients may lead to increased intracellular concentrations of lithium, and this may explain toxic reactions at serum lithium levels well within the maintenance range (0.5 to 1.0 mEq/liter).

Answers

1. (B)
2. (B and D)
3. (A, B, and C)
4. (B)
5. (A)↓
   (B)↓
   (C)↓
   (D)↓
   (E)↑
6. (B)
7. (E)
8. (A)
9. (E)

References

1. Hicks, R., *et al.*: The pharmacokinetics of psychotropic medication in the elderly: A review. *Journal of Clinical Psychiatry*, 43: 347–385, 1981.
2. Schou, M.: Lithium in psychiatric therapy and prophylaxis. *Journal of Psychiatric Training and Research*, 6: 69–95, 1968.
3. Schou, M.: Pharmacology and toxocology of lithium. *Annual Review of Pharmacology and Toxicology*, 16: 231–243, 1976.
4. Ayd, F.: Guidelines for the use of lithium in the elderly. *International Drug Therapy Newsletter*, 17(6): 1982.

5. Raskind, M. A. and Eisdorfer, C.: Psychopharmacology of the aged. In: *Drug Treatment of Mental Disorders* (ed.: G. Simpson). Raven Press, New York, 1975.
6. Ban, T. (ed.): *Psychopharmacology for the Aged*. S. Karger, Basel/New York, 1980.

CASE 38: PREMENSTRUAL SYNDROME IN A 35-YEAR-OLD WOMAN

Mrs. R. is a 35-year-old mother of three who presents with the chief complaint that "Something has to be done about my cycles, I can't stand it any more." The patient goes on to explain that she has been seen by her internist over the past few years for marked physical and emotional difficulties relative to her menstrual periods. She states that her difficulties have become so severe that at present they jeopardize many aspects of her interpersonal life, including her relationship with her husband and children. They also are causing her increasing vocational difficulties. She says that on the sixth day prior to her menses she develops a number of symptoms, including dysphoria, anxiety and tension, irritability, and hostility. At times she becomes obsessed with eating sweets, and frequently also has many somatic complaints. These include pain in her breasts and abdomen, bloating and edema, and headaches which can be extremely severe. These prevent her from going to work, which consists of a major role in a marketing firm. She states that on one or two occasions she has even noticed that she has had minor car accidents because of general feelings of perplexity and preoccupation during the premenstrual period.

1. The incidence of women who have severe premenstrual symptoms leading to medical or psychiatric intervention is about:
   A. 5%
   B. 50%
   C. 80%
2. The diagnosis of premenstrual syndrome should be based on:
   A. Specific symptom clusters
   B. Affective liability

C. Timing
D. A and C

Discussion

At least 20% and as many as 80% of all women report mild to moderate mood or somatic changes premenstrually. It is estimated that 5% seek medical or psychiatric treatment as a consequence of these symptoms interfering with normal functioning. A myriad of nonspecific and specific symptoms have been reported premenstrually. However, this condition is not diagnosed by specific symptom clusters, but rather by its timing.

3. The drug of choice for the treatment of premenstrual syndrome is:
   A. Progesterone
   B. Placebo
   C. Antidepressants
   D. Diuretics
   E. None of the above
4. In the event that serious depressive symptoms occur, the drug category of choice is:
   A. Lithium carbonate
   B. Tricyclic antidepressants
   C. Major tranquilizers
   D. Benzodiazepines

Discussion

No specific agent has been shown to be effective in alleviating premenstrual tension. Placebo-induced improvement has occurred at a rate of as high as 60% in some studies. Significant edema can be treated with diuretics, although these drugs do not *per se* specifically help to improve a negative affect. No replicated, well-controlled studies have unequivocally confirmed that any one treatment is preferable to any other for the premenstrual syndrome. For the treatment of women with affective (i.e., depressive) disorders who experience premenstrual exacerbations, the psychiatrist should consider using a tricyclic antidepressant. Lithium carbonate has been used in many patients with affective symptoms.

Answers

1. (A)
2. (D)
3. (E)
4. (B)

References

1. Hamilton, J. A., *et al.*: Premenstrual mood changes: A guide to evaluation and treatment. *Psychiatric Annals*, 14(6): 426–435, 1984.
2. Janowsky, D. S.: Menstrual and premenstrual mood disorders. In: *Phenomenology and Treatment of Psychophysiological Disorders* (ed.: W. E. Fann). Spectrum Publications, New York, 1982.
3. Greene, J.: Recent trends in treatment of premenstrual syndrome: A critical review. In: *Behavior and the Menstrual Cycle* (ed.: R. C. Friedman). Marcel Dekker, New York, 1982.
4. Sampson, G. A.: Premenstrual syndrome: A double blind controlled trial of progesterone and placebo. *British Journal of Psychiatry*, 135: 209–215, 1979.

SECTION III
NEUROTIC DISORDERS

CASE 39: TREATMENT OF SITUATIONAL ANXIETY

The patient is a 22-year-old woman with no prior psychiatric history. She comes to you complaining of insomnia and a high level of anxiety caused by her marital problems, which began approximately a month ago. She was referred by her internist, who had done a thorough medical workup and found nothing abnormal. Your mental status examination is normal, with the exception of some depression and anxiety related mainly to her recent stresses.

1. Correct statements about the assessment of the patient's anxiety, with regard to the use of antianxiety medications are:
   A. There are good methods available for analyzing the type and intensity of anxiety in an objective manner
   B. Anxiety will usually improve with time alone
   C. The patient's history is fairly consistent with major depressive disorder, and thus antidepressant medications are strongly indicated
   D. There are different meanings to and different prognoses for anxiety, depending on an individual's sex, age, marital status, and social class

Discussion

There are a number of reasons why it is difficult to evaluate the effectiveness of minor tranquilizers in the treatment of anxiety. As discussed by Greenblatt and Shader in *Benzodiazepines in Clinical Practice*, anxiety is frequently a self-limited process, often improving with time alone. Thus, any medication may appear effective in the treatment of this somewhat ephemeral disorder. In addition, good research is hampered by the lack of techniques for objectively measuring levels of anxiety. The case presented here is not at all consistent with primary affective disorder. The symptoms of primary affective disorder usually include psychological feelings of hopelessness, worthlessness, and uselessness, along with sadness, bodily symptoms of anorexia and insomnia. Anxiety can be a symptom of a depressive disorder, but the underlying affective syndrome is usually fairly obvious. Thus, anxiety must be considered in the context of the total clinical picture, and not just as a treatable syndrome.

2. In choosing a drug to alleviate the stresses of everyday life, one should consider the following areas of potential harm:
   A. The physician may obscure the source of the problem and thus bury an area of further abnormalities by prescribing medications too early
   B. Almost all drugs used to treat anxiety are potential drugs of abuse
   C. The physician may interfere with a patient's chance for personal growth by beginning medications prematurely
   D. There is a high risk of severe side effects from most minor tranquilizers

Discussion

Anxiety is a normal reaction to stress. Thus, the physician must guard against reacting too quickly by prescribing minor tranquilizers such as chlordiazepoxide (Librium) and diazepam (Valium). In addition, in administering these drugs, one should recognize that there are potential risks. While the incidence of severe side effects is relatively low, most of these drugs have a potential for abuse, habituation, and addiction. Psychological dependence is probably quite common, and a number of cases of physical dependence have been reported.

3. You decide to use an antianxiety drug and are guided by the following statements:
   A. Oxazepam (Serax) should be considered because it is not addicting
   B. Meprobamate (Miltown) should be considered, primarily because it has a lower frequency of side effects than other antianxiety drugs

C. Chlordiazepoxide (Librium) should be used before diazepam (Valium) because it is less addicting
D. Benzodiazopines are preferable to other sedative–hypnotics, such as barbiturates

Discussion

There is little indication that any one of the benzodiazepine medications is superior in effectiveness to the others. The choice of a specific medication depends on an understanding of the medication's side effects, not its relative usefulness. All of the antianxiety drugs are potentially physiologically addicting. Meprobamate has a similar, if not greater, incidence of side effects than the other minor tranquilizers, and is also felt to be less effective, to have a greater abuse liability, and to more commonly produce serious poisoning in overdoses than occurs with the benzodiazepines. The barbiturates cause more respiratory depression and have a higher addiction potential, and are not indicated in the treatment of anxiety disorders. There are no major differences between chlordiazepoxide and diazepam in terms of efficacy.

4. Correct statements about the general properties of the benzodiazepines include:
   A. The central antianxiety effects of these drugs are probably related to their effects on the limbic system
   B. These drugs have been shown to have muscle-relaxing properties in both animals and humans
   C. These drugs have been shown to have anticonvulsant properties in both animals and humans
   D. Studies have demonstrated that no more than 5% of medical patients receive one of these drugs

Discussion

Antianxiety drugs are used extensively in our society, with an estimated one-third of all adults having used some type of antianxiety agent. The benzodiazepines have strong anticonvulsant properties in addition to their antianxiety properties. The mode of action of the benzodiazepines is not completely understood, but most of their actions are felt to occur in the central nervous system, and attempts to localize the site of their activity have implicated the limbic system.

5. Correct statements about the administration of benzodiazepines include:
   A. Rapid intravenous infusion of these drugs has been very uncommonly shown to cause transient bradycardia, hypotension, or apnea
   B. Peak blood levels from intramuscular injection of these drugs are generally reached at erratic intervals
   C. These drugs generally cause much less circulatory and respiratory depression than is true of the barbiturates
   D. Peak blood levels from oral doses of diazepam and chlordiazepoxide are generally reached in about 6 hours

Discussion

Blood levels from single intramuscular doses of chlordiazepoxide are lower and peak later than when the dose is given by mouth. Peak concentrations after oral ingestion occur at approximately 1½ hours. Intramuscular injections peak between 90 minutes and 10 hours. Benzodiazepines have been given intravenously for a number of diagnostic and treatment procedures, and generally have been assumed to be quite safe, with injection-site complications the most common problems observed. Thus, serious symptoms such as bradycardia, hypotension, or apnea are unlikely to be seen, although they have been reported.

Answers

1. (B and D)
2. (A, B, and C)
3. (D)
4. (A, B, and C)
5. (A, B, and C)

References

1. Greenblatt, D. J. and Shader, R. I.: *Benzodiazepines in Clinical Practice.* Raven Press, New York, 1974.

2. Greenblatt, D. J. and Shader, R. I.: Medical intelligence, drug therapy, benzodiazepines (first of two parts). *New England Journal of Medicine*, 291(19): 1011–1015, 1974.
3. Greenblatt, D. J. and Shader, R. I.: Medical intelligence, drug therapy, benzodiazepines (second of two parts). *New England Journal of Medicine*, 291(20): 1239–1243, 1974.
4. Blackwell, B.: Psychotropic drugs in use today. *Journal of the American Medical Association*, 225: 1637–1641, 1973.
5. Hussey, H. H.: Drugs for anxiety. *Journal of the American Medical Association*, 228: 875, 1974.
6. Greenblatt, D. J., Shader, R. I., and Koch-Weser, J.: Slow absorption of intramuscular chlordiazepoxide. *New England Journal of Medicine*, 291: 1116–1118, 1974.
7. Rickels, K.: Benzodiazepines in the treatment of anxiety. *American Journal of Psychotherapy*, 36: 358–370, 1982.
8. Cohen, S.: The benzodiazepines. *Psychiatric Annals*, 131: 65–70, 1983.
9. Mavissakalian, M.: Pharmacologic treatment of anxiety disorders. *Journal of Clinical Psychiatry*, 43: 487–491, 1982.

CASE 40: TREATMENT OF RECURRENT PANIC ATTACKS

Mr. R. is a 42-year-old married white man who works as a city administrator. He has requested a consultation for treatment of his panic attacks. He describes a long history of having periods of extreme uneasiness, consisting of sweating, an ever-fearful feeling, a fast heart rate, a tight feeling in his chest, occasional hyperventilation, and a feeling of dread when confined in closed-in places, such as elevators or restaurants. Between episodes, which have occurred approximately once per week, the patient reports having felt mildly to moderately anxious, but able to function well. The patient had previously been treated for his panic attacks and anxiety with diazepam (Valium) 5 to 10 mg every 4 to 6 hours. He had been carefully evaluated to rule out the possibility that anxiety-producing medical factors were causing his symptoms. Routine laboratory tests and a physical examination were normal. The patient discontinued his diazepam approximately 3 months before his consultation with you.

1. Medical conditions that can mimic severe anxiety include:
   A. Hyperthyroidism
   B. Pheochromocytoma
   C. Temporal-lobe epilepsy
   D. Hypoglycemia
   E. All of the above
   F. None of the above
2. Diazepam:
   A. Is effective in the treatment of panic attacks
   B. Has little effectiveness in treating panic attacks
3. Useful in the treatment of panic attacks is (are):
   A. Monoamine oxidase inhibitors
   B. Desipramine
   C. Imipramine
   D. Alprazolam
   E. None of the above
   F. All of the above

Discussion

Tricyclic antidepressants and monoamine oxidase inhibitors (MAOIs) are being used to alleviate panic-attack symptoms and anxiety in patients without evidence of depression. Major drugs noted to exert this antipanic effect include desipramine (Norpramin), imipramine (Tofranil), phenelzine (Nardil), and alprazolam (Xanax).

Case Continued: On the basis of the patient's history, it was decided that a trial of desipramine was indicated as treatment for the panic attacks. A dose of 25 mg per day orally was increased to 75 mg per day over a period of 1 week, and to 100 mg per day 3 days later. Since the patient lived in a distant city, without local psychiatrists available, it was decided that once his medication was stabilized, a local family physician would monitor the medication.

4. In the treatment of panic attacks, the optimal dose of desipramine is often:
   A. Less than that required for the treatment of major depressive disorders

B. The same as that required for the treatment of major depressive disorders
C. More than that required for the treatment of major depressive disorders

Discussion

The doses of antidepressant drug effective in alleviating panic attacks can be relatively low as compared to those needed to alleviate depression. Furthermore, the time course of symptom alleviation is often considerably longer than that required when depression is being treated.

Case Continued: After 2 weeks of taking desipramine, the patient stated that he felt slightly more relaxed. He was seen at 2-week intervals over the next 1½ months, and by the end of the second month of treatment was much improved, having almost no serious panic attacks. However, he also continued to avoid elevators and restaurants because he feared that he might have an attack.

5. If a residual anticipatory anxiety exists following the alleviation of panic attacks by a tricyclic antidepressant or monoamine oxidase inhibitor, the preferred treatment(s) is (are):
   A. A higher dose of antidepressant drug
   B. A benzodiazepine such as diazepam or chlordiazepoxide
   C. Propranolol
   D. B and C
   E. A and B

Case Continued: To combat the patient's anticipatory anxiety over the possibility of having another panic attack, it was decided to begin a trial of diazepam at low dosage. Diazepam was therefore prescribed at a dose of 5 mg every 4 to 6 hours as needed when the patient was contemplating going into a closed area. Administration of the diazepam to combat the fear of having another panic attack, plus desipramine to alleviate the panic attacks, and psychological support and behavioral deconditioning allowed the patient to function with minimal uneasiness over the subsequent year, during which time the diazepam was tapered slowly and eventually stopped as the patient became less and less fearful of having another attack.

Discussion

Although a tricyclic antidepressant can effectively alleviate the symptoms of a panic attack, such a drug is not as effective in alleviating the anxiety and fear that a panic attack might occur in the future. Such fear may lead to a constriction of activity and function. A classic antianxiety agent, such as diazepam or chlordiazepoxide, can be effective in treating this "anticipatory anxiety."

Answers

1. (F)
2. (A)
3. (F)
4. (A)
5. (B)

References

1. Rickels, K.: Benzodiazepines in the treatment of anxiety. *American Journal of Psychotherapy*, 36: 358–370, 1982.
2. Shader, R. I., Goodman, M., and Gever, J.: Panic disorders: Current perspectives. *Journal of Clinical Psychopharmacology*, 2 (Supplement): 2S–26S, 1982.
3. Mavissakalian, N.: Pharmacologic treatment of anxiety disorders. *Journal of Clinical Psychiatry*, 43: 487–491, 1982.
4. Cohen, S.: The benzodiazepines. *Psychiatric Annals*, 131: 65–70, 1983.
5. Zitrin, C. M., Klein, D. F., Woerner, M. G., and Ross, D. C.: Treatment of phobias: I. Comparison of imipramine hydrochloride and placebo. *Archives of General Psychiatry*, 40: 125–138, 1983.
6. Sheehan, D. B., Ballenger, J., and Jacobsen, G.: Treatment of phobic anxiety with phobic, hysterical and hypochondriacal symptoms. *Archives of General Psychiatry*, 37: 51–59, 1980.
7. Hoehn-Saric, R., Merchant, A., Keyse, M., and Smith, V.: Effects of clonidine on anxiety disorders. *Archives of General Psychiatry*, 38: 1278–1282, 1981.
8. Aden, G. C.: Alprazolam in clinically anxious patients with depressed moods. *Journal of Clinical Psychiatry*, 44: 22–24, 1983.

CASE 41: TREATMENT OF ANXIETY WITH ANTIANXIETY AGENTS

The patient is a 35-year-old white male who gives a history of severe anxiety attacks, characterized by palpitations, sweating, hyperventilation, numbness and tingling of the hands and feet, and muscle pains—all in episodes lasting 5 to 20 minutes and occurring once or twice a week. These episodes have occurred since the patient was in his middle to late 20s. He comes to see you requesting medications to help him with his problem.

1. You consider using benzodiazepines. In choosing between specific drugs you are guided by the following correct statements:
   A. One must beware of oxazepam (Serax), because it tends to accumulate in the body with repeated doses
   B. If oxazepam is chosen, it can easily be given in a once-daily dose
   C. There is no evidence that oxazepam is either more or less effective than the other benzodiazepines in treating anxiety

Discussion

The pharmacokinetics of oxazepam are quite different from those of other benzodiazepines. Its half-life is between 3 and 21 hours, with a mean of around 4 to 15 hours. Unlike diazepam (Valium) or chlordiazepoxide (Librium), this drug does not accumulate in the body with repeated doses. At present there is no evidence that oxazepam is either more effective or less effective than any of the other benzodiazepines, such as chlordiazepoxide or diazepam.

2. You consider the use of diazepam. Correct statements about this drug include:
   A. Its active metabolite tends to accumulate in the body with repeated doses
   B. The drug must be given in three to four divided daily doses in order to be effective
   C. Major active metabolites tend to remain in the bloodstream longer than diazepam itself

D. If toxic effects were not seen at a given dose level after 2 days, they will probably not be encountered

Discussion

Diazepam is a lipid-soluble (and relatively water-insoluble) substance that binds strongly to serum albumin. The half-life of this drug is relatively long (anywhere from 20 to 50 hours), with some of the active metabolites remaining in the body longer than the parent drug itself. Thus, toxic effects can occur with accumulation of the drug, and after a steady-state blood level is reached. Some authors feel it is not necessary to give the drug in divided doses.

3. Correct statements about the use of antianxiety agents in an anxiety state include:
   A. There is good evidence that the benzodiazepines are superior to placebo in the treatment of acute anxiety
   B. There is some indication that the benzodiazepines, if given in the first 6 weeks of pregnancy, are associated with an increase in fetal malformations
   C. The side effect of central-nervous-system depression by antianxiety agents is probably more severe in elderly patients or patients with low serum albumin levels
   D. There is good evidence that the benzodiazepines are better than a placebo in treating chronic anxiety

Discussion

Most trials comparing a benzodiazepine to placebo show a clear superiority of the active drug in the treatment of acute anxiety. However, there is limited evidence that the benzodiazepines are effective in the treatment of chronic anxiety. Side effects of the benzodiazepines are relatively benign; excessive central nervous system depression is the most common side effect—one that is usually dose dependent and more likely to occur in elderly persons. In addition, there is some indication that prescribing of chlordiazepoxide or other benzodiazepines in early pregnancy may rarely result in an elevated rate of fetal anomalies.

4. Correct statements about the disorders in which the benzodiazepines have been shown to be effective include:
   A. They are definitely effective as antipsychotic agents in schizophrenia
   B. They are effective in relieving psychomotor retardation in neurotic disorders
   C. They are effective in relieving status epilepsy in psychomotor and myoclonic disorders

Discussion

The disorders for which the benzodiazepines have been shown to be effective are quite limited, with acute anxiety, seizure disorder, and the treatment of alcoholic withdrawal leading the list. These drugs are also useful in the induction of anesthesia, for cardioversion, and for endoscopy. The benzodiazepines are usually not effective in the treatment of schizophrenia or depression, or in the prevention of recurrence of anxiety attacks.

5. Correct statements about complications from the administration of the benzodiazepines include:
   A. Benzodiazepines can produce paradoxical excitement in some patients
   B. Phlebitis has been reported in over 3% of patients receiving benzodiazepines intravenously
   C. The potential for a fatal outcome with an overdose of these drugs is a good deal less than for most other sedative–hypnotic drugs
   D. These drugs can be safely administered with oral anticoagulants

Discussion

Among the complications reported for benzodiazepines, paradoxical excitement and the possibility of an increase in depression or self-destructive behavior has been noted. Phlebitis has been reported in about 3½% of patients receiving these drugs intravenously. The addiction potential of these drugs is considerably less than for the other sedative–hypnotic medications, and the potential for a lethal overdose is a great deal less than with other sedative drugs. The benzodiazepines, unlike the barbiturates, usually do not cause clinically important microsomal enzyme induction. Other side effects, such as hepatotoxicity, have been reported anecdotally in only a few cases.

Answers

1. (C)
2. (A and C)
3. (A, B, and C)
4. (C)
5. (A, B, C, and D)

References

1. Greenblatt, D. J. and Shader, R. I.: Medical intelligence, drug therapy, benzodiazepines. *New England Journal of Medicine*, 291(19): 1011–1015, 1974.
2. Milkovich, L. and van den Berg, B. J.: Effects of prenatal meprobamate and chlordiazepoxide hydrochloride on human embryonic and fetal development. *New England Journal of Medicine*, 291: 1268–1271, 1974.
3. Shader, R. I. and Greenblatt, D. J.: Clinical implications of benzodiazepine pharmacokinetics. *American Journal of Psychiatry*, 134(6): 652–656, 1977.
4. Aden, G. C.: Alprazolam in clinically anxious patients with depressed minds. *Journal of Clinical Psychiatry*, 44: 22–24, 1983.
5. Kalian, M. M.: Pharmacologic treatment of anxiety disorders. *Journal of Clinical Psychiatry*, 43: 487–491, 1982.
6. Rickels, K.: Benzodiazepines in the treatment of anxiety. *American Journal of Psychotherapy*, 36: 358–370, 1982.
7. Mavissakalian, M.: Pharmacologic treatment of anxiety disorders. *Journal of Clinical Psychiatry*, 43: 487–491, 1982.
8. Cohen, S.: The benzodiazepines. *Psychiatric Annals*, 131: 65–70, 1983.
9. Sheehan, D. V., Ballenger, J., and Jacobsen, G.: Treatment of phobic anxiety with phobic, hysterical and hypochondriacal symptoms. *Archives of General Psychiatry*, 37: 51–59, 1980.

CASE 42: TREATMENT OF ANXIETY WITH PROPRANOLOL

You are asked to consult in the case of a 35-year-old electrical engineer who complains of anxiety attacks. His physician has done a thorough basic medical examination and found nothing wrong. The patient asks to see a psychiatrist because he has heard about a "miracle drug" called propranolol for the treatment of anxiety. You review the patient's history, perform a mental-status examination, gather information from family members, and arrive at the diagnosis of generalized anxiety disorder. The physician asks your advice on the use of propranolol.

1. Correct statements about the actions of propranolol include:
   A. Propranolol blocks beta-adrenergic receptors, which are most commonly seen in the heart, skeletal muscle, blood vessels, and bronchial muscles
   B. Propranolol works equally as well on alpha- and beta-adrenergic receptors
   C. Propranolol blocks the increase in the heart rate and dilation of skeletal-muscle blood vessels that usually occurs with beta-adrenergic stimulation
   D. Propranolol blocks receptors that are uniformly most sensitive to norepinephrine

Discussion

Propranolol is a beta-adrenergic blocking drug that affects nerve receptors responsive to isoproterenol (beta-receptors), and has less effect on norepinephrine-responsive alpha-receptors. Beta-receptors are found in greatest abundance in the heart, skeletal muscle, blood vessels, bronchial musculature, digestive tract, bladder, and ciliary muscles. Beta stimulation usually results in an increase in heart rate and myocardial contraction, and in bronchodilation. The beta-blocking agents become bound to receptor sites competitively with isoproterenol, and are also felt to stabilize membranes.

2. Among the effects of propranolol on the central nervous system are that:
   A. This drug crosses the blood–brain barrier
   B. Its actions in the brain could be independent of beta blockade
   C. The use of this drug for psychiatric disorders is common but still considered experimental
   D. Part of the mechanism of action of this drug could be related to a stabilization of cell membranes

Discussion

Propranolol crosses the blood–brain barrier and exhibits actions on the brain that may be independent of its beta-blocking effects (such as central-nervous-system depression).

3. In relation to propranolol's use in the treatment of anxiety, one can cite:
   A. That propranolol has been shown to be effective in blocking the anxiety seen in thyrotoxicosis
   B. That propranolol is especially good for anxiety states accompanied by physical symptoms of anxiety
   C. That this drug has not been shown to be superior to diazepam (Valium) in the treatment of anxiety
   D. That this drug is especially good for the treatment of chronic anxiety
4. Statements which characterize the use of propranolol in the treatment of psychiatric disorders include:
   A. Only uncontrolled studies have shown this drug to be dramatically useful in the treatment of psychosis
   B. The drug has been shown to block the depressant effect of alcohol in humans
   C. Repeated controlled studies have shown this drug to block the euphoric effects of heroin
5. Properties of propranolol that should be considered before its use is begun include:
   A. Toxic doses of this drug have been shown to produce cardiac arrhythmias
   B. Hypoglycemia has occurred in association with this drug
   C. Toxic psychoses may be associated with this drug
   D. A drug-induced depression has been reported in association with propranolol administration.

Discussion

Propranolol has been shown to be effective in blocking the anxiety seen in thyrotoxicosis, and has been useful in the control of hypertension. Its usefulness as a drug in psychiatry is probably limited to acute anxiety states and functional cardiac disorders, such as anxiety neurosis. It has also been recommended for use in the treatment of psychosis, alcoholism and alcoholic withdrawal, heroin addiction, and amphetamine toxicity—but none of these has proven to be justified by controlled studies. For acute anxiety, propranolol has not been shown to be superior to minor tranquilizers. Adverse reactions to this medication include cardiovascular problems, such as pulmonary edema or congestive heart failure, and changes in blood pressure and respiratory function, hypoglycemia, toxic psychosis, and depression.

Answers

1. (A and C)
2. (A, B, C, and D)
3. (A, B, and C)
4. (A)
5. (A, B, C, and D)

Reference

1. Jefferson, J. W.: Beta-adrenergic receptor blocking drugs in psychiatry. *Archives of General Psychiatry*, 31: 681–691, 1974.

CASE 43: EVALUATION AND TREATMENT OF INSOMNIA

The patient is a 52-year-old woman whom you treated 2 years ago for marital conflict. At that time, no major psychopathology was present, and the treatment was terminated after five visits. The patient now calls complaining of insomnia and asking for some sleep medications.

1. The differential diagnosis (diagnoses) of probable causes of insomnia in this case include(s):
   A. Major depressive disorder
   B. Schizophrenia
   C. Drug abuse
   D. A and C

Discussion

Insomnia should not be considered a disease, but rather a symptom—one that can be seen in a wide variety of disorders. There are a number of syndromes that can present with insomnia as the major symptom. These include sleep apnea, narcolepsy, night terrors, somnambulism, the restless leg syndrome, nocturnal myoclonus, and idiopathic insomnia. In addition, insomnia can be seen as a symptom of a number of major and minor psychiatric disorders—especially affective disorders, drug abuse, and alcoholism. While schizophrenia can present with a sleep disorder, this diagnosis would probably not fit the patient previously described.

2. Correct statements about what should be done at this point in your evaluation include:
   A. A more thorough history should be taken about possible psychiatric symptoms
   B. The patient should be asked to list all medications that she is now taking
   C. A history of the patient's drinking practices is required
   D. A 2-week supply of sleep medication should be given over the phone and the patient brought in to see you on a routine basis in 2 weeks

Discussion

It is a grave mistake to treat insomnia as a primary diagnosis. Such a practice usually leads to the prescription of sedative-hypnotic medications without adequately evaluating the patient. The first approach to evaluating a patient with insomnia is to acquire a complete medical history and do a thorough psychiatric evaluation, making special note of any medications or drugs of abuse that the patient may be taking. Special care must be taken to evaluate the drinking history. Drug or alcohol abuse can severely disturb normal sleeping patterns.

3. An evaluation of the patient reveals no obvious psychiatric pathology and you are called on to treat the insomnia as a disorder, rather than

as a symptom of a major psychiatric disease. At this point, the differential diagnosis includes:
A. Nocturnal myoclonus
B. Restless leg syndrome
C. Sleep apnea
D. Narcolepsy

Discussion

Nocturnal myoclonus is characterized by pronounced jerks, which may rhythmically occur in both legs simultaneously. The jerking may be pronounced enough to arouse the patient from sleep. The restless leg syndrome is usually characterized by a feeling that there is something crawling inside the legs. This sensation occurs during the day—perhaps each hour or two—as well as during sleep. Moving about banishes the symptoms, and at night the patient must get out of bed and walk around before he can go back to sleep. Sleep apnea is characterized by the inability to breathe while asleep. Thus the night is characterized by a series of awakenings, with great restlessness as the patient comes out of sleep every several minutes in order to breathe. Narcolepsy and other hypersomnic states can be thought by patients to be a form of insomnia. All of these disorders must be considered in the evaluation of insomnia.

4. The patient asks about taking over-the-counter sleep medications. Correct statements about these drugs include:
A. Most contain bromides
B. These drugs have been shown in controlled studies to be effective hypnotics
C. These drugs produce a natural, sequential, sleep pattern
D. Most of these drugs contain scopolamine-like substances

Discussion

Over-the-counter sleep medications usually contain a belladonna alkaloid. Scopolamine, in therapeutic doses, can cause drowsiness, euphoria, amnesia, fatigue, and a dreamless sleep. However, the same doses occasionally cause excitement, restlessness, hallucinations, or delusions. It is unlikely that these drugs are effective hypnotics, but accurate studies of their effectiveness have not been carried out.

5. The proper evaluation of sleep disorders includes:
   A. A thorough psychiatric evaluation
   B. A good physical examination
   C. A sleep-laboratory evaluation for patients whose insomnia is chronic
   D. A supplementary history taken from the spouse or others close to the patient

Discussion

As the discussions above would indicate, a complaint of insomnia should not be met with the automatic prescription of sleep medications. Every patient with insomnia requires a good physical examination, a thorough psychiatric evaluation, and a careful history taken from an ancillary person, such as the spouse. For those patients with severe insomnia or chronic complaints of sleeplessness, a sleep-laboratory evaluation should be done.

Answers

1. (D)
2. (A, B, and C)
3. (A, B, C, and D)
4. (D)
5. (A, B, C, and D)

References

1. Dement, W. C. and Guilleminault, C.: Sleep disorders: The state of the art. *Hospital Practice*, 8: 57–71, 1973.
2. Dement, W. C.: *Some Must Watch while Some Must Sleep*. Stanford Alumnae Association, Stanford, CA, 1972, pp. 73–93.
3. Ullman, K. C. and Groh, R. H.: Identification in treatment of acute psychotic states, secondary to the usage of over-the-counter sleeping preparations. *American Journal of Psychiatry*, 128: 1244–1248, 1972.

4. Allen, R. M.: Attenuation of drug-induced anxiety dreams and pavor nocturnus by benzodiazepines. *Journal of Clinical Psychiatry*, 44: 106–108, 1983.
5. Lader, M.: Insomnia and short-acting benzodiazepine hypnotics. *Journal of Clinical Psychiatry*, 44: 47–53, 1983.
6. Gillin, J. C., Duncan, W., Pettigrew, K. D., Frankel, B. L., and Snyder, F.: Successful separation of depressed and insomniac subjects by EEG sleep data. *Archives of General Psychiatry*, 36: 85–90, 1979.
7. Kupfer, D. J., Spiker, D. G., Coble, P. A., *et al.*: Sleep and treatment prediction in endogenous depression. *American Journal of Psychiatry*, 138: 429–434, 1981.

CASE 44: CHRONIC INSOMNIA AND ITS TREATMENT

A 48-year-old woman who was previously being evaluated for insomnia disappears from treatment. Eighteen months later she again comes for treatment, complaining of insomnia. She reports that she has been taking three secobarbital (Seconal) pills at night for the last 8 months. Her insomnia continues.

1. Controlled studies have revealed which of the following?
   A. Hypnotic effectiveness disappears after 2 weeks to 1 month
   B. All hypnotics are basically alike in their effect on sleep patterns
   C. Almost all hypnotics are physiologically addicting
   D. All major hypnotics are essentially alike in effectiveness
2. It is decided that the secobarbital will be stopped. Correct statements about the best procedure for and effects of stopping this drug include:
   A. It is best that the patient be withdrawn from the drug quickly. Since she is not physically addicted, the termination of her psychological dependence should be as rapid as possible
   B. When the secobarbital is stopped, the patient can expect to experience an increased frequency and intensity of dreams
   C. The patient can expect relatively smooth sleep (that is, no fragmentation of sleep) within a few days after stopping the drug
   D. The patient can expect to have even greater difficulty falling asleep once the drug is stopped

Discussion

Despite the fact that hypnotic drugs have been reported to be effective, most patients with insomnia complain of persistent and severe sleeplessness, even after chronic use of multiple doses of these drugs. Kales and his co-authors discussed a series of 10 patients who had been using hypnotics for periods ranging from months to years. A sleep-laboratory comparison with insomniac controls who were not receiving medication demonstrated a significant decrease of rapid-eye-movement (REM) sleep in the chronic hypnotic users. A striking finding was that the drug-using patients had as great or greater difficulty in falling asleep, staying asleep or both as the insomniac controls who were not using medication—a finding apparent within 2 weeks to a month of beginning the regular use of hypnotics. Abrupt withdrawal of the ineffective drug was not recommended, due to psychological and physiological changes that contribute to a drug-withdrawal insomnia and hypnotic-drug dependence. The ineffectiveness of hypnotic drugs demonstrated in the Kales study indicates the need for changes in guidelines for evaluating and advertising hypnotic drugs. There are a number of different hypnotic medications with differing abilities to suppress specific sleep stages and ease the induction of sleep. However, almost all hypnotics are physiologically addicting.

3. L-Tryptophan is considered for use as a hypnotic. Correct statements about this drug include:
   A. It is effective as a "natural" hypnotic
   B. Its effect probably is peripheral since it does not cross the blood–brain barrier
   C. In doses as low as 1 g at bedtime, it significantly reduces sleep latency
   D. L-Tryptophan causes little or no interference with sleep stages

Discussion

L-Tryptophan is probably a naturally occurring hypnotic that rapidly crosses the blood–brain barrier. If given in doses of 1 g, the result usually is a decrease in sleep latency with little disturbance of sleep stages.

4. A good nonmedicinal approach to insomnia includes:
   A. Stopping all medications that could possibly interfere with sleep
   B. Stopping all caffeinated drinks throughout the day
   C. Stopping drinking alcoholic beverages
   D. Putting the patient on a fairly rigid schedule of bedtimes
5. A good procedure for treating a patient who complains of insomnia despite taking three secobarbital tablets nightly for the last year includes:
   A. The drug dose should immediately be cut to one pill nightly
   B. Another barbiturate hypnotic should be instituted
   C. The patient should be hospitalized for a course of detoxification
   D. The patient should be warned to expect vivid dreams or nightmares
6. Insomnia is a major consequence of chronic alcohol ingestion:
   A. True
   B. False

Discussion

In evaluating the insomniac patient, the following figures should be kept in mind: approximately 40% of patients who complain of insomnia lose sleep because of drug dependence; about 10% have sleep apnea; about 20% suffer from psychiatric disorders; and the remaining 30% have idiopathic insomnia. If the patient is dependent upon hypnotics, Kales *et al.* recommend the following procedure: the hypnotic should be withdrawn very gradually, at the rate of one therapeutic dose every 5 or 6 days. The patient should be told that changes, including increased dreaming, vivid dreams, and nightmares may occur; and another hypnotic, such as flurazepam (Dalmane) may have to be instituted. However, it is preferable to use no ancillary drug if at all possible. In attempting a nonmedicinal approach to insomnia, the following suggestions are indicated: counseling and reassurance along with instructions on how to relax, how to avoid disturbing physical or mental activity before sleep, and how to choose a bedtime suited to individual characteristics. In addition, medications that may interfere with sleep and caffeinated drinks should be stopped, as should the intake of alcohol. The patient may be put on a fairly rigid schedule of bedtimes and awakenings. Insomnia is a major consequence of chronic alcohol ingestion, and may be considered to be a drug-dependent insomnia. A history of alcohol use should be explored in all insomnia patients.

Answers

1. (A and C)
2. (B and D)
3. (A, C, and D)
4. (A, B, C, and D)
5. (D)
6. (A)

References

1. Dement, W. C. and Guilleminault, C.: Sleep disorders: The state of the art. *Hospital Practice*, 8: 57–71, 1973.
2. Dement, W. C.: *Some Must Watch while Some Must Sleep*. Stanford Alumnae Association, Stanford, CA, 1972, pp. 73–93.
3. Ullman, K. C. and Groh, R. H.: Identification and treatment of acute psychotic states, secondary to the usage of over-the-counter sleeping preparations. *American Journal of Psychiatry*, 128: 1244–1248, 1972.
4. Hartman, E.: L-Tryptophan: A possible natural hypnotic substance (Editorial). *Journal of the American Medical Association*, 230: 1680–1681, 1974.
5. Lader, M.: Insomnia and short-acting benzodiazepine hypnotics. *Journal of Clinical Psychiatry*, 44: 47–53, 1983.

SECTION IV
ORGANIC BRAIN SYNDROME

CASE 45: TREATMENT OF ACUTE-ONSET ORGANIC BRAIN SYNDROME

A 62-year-old man is in good health and has no psychiatric problems until 48 hours after routine prostatic surgery, when he becomes confused and agitated. A psychiatric consultant is called. A mental-status examination reveals an agitated, confused, difficult-to-handle patient who is disoriented to time and place as well as person. He is afraid that the nurses are trying to poison him and convinced he will not leave the hospital alive.

1. Correct statements about evaluating this patient include:
   A. A first step should involve a review of the patient's physical status
   B. A first step should involve contacting the family to determine the stresses under which the man was functioning prior to surgery
   C. A first step should include a review of all medications that the patient has been taking
   D. A first step should involve the prescription of major tranquilizers

Discussion

The patient is suffering from a confusional state of acute onset and has an organic brain syndrome. This diagnosis is based primarily on a mental-status examination and is usually applied to patients with recognizable medical and neurological disorders affecting brain structure and function. The diagnosis depends on finding impairment of orientation, memory, and other intellectual function, in addition to other psychiatric symptoms which may occur, including hallucinations, delusions, depression, obsessions, and personality change. Judgment is impaired, and the patient may not be aware of the disorder. Correction of the underlying medical and//or neurological condition is the principal aim of therapy. Two problems which frequently cause an organic brain syndrome are withdrawal from, adverse reaction to, or receiving toxic doses of medications; or a metabolic imbalance; or both. Psychotropic drugs should not be used for treating this disorder until an attempt has been made to establish the cause of the organic brain syndrome.

2. The incidence of organic brain syndrome after surgery increases with:
   A. Increasing age
   B. A prior history of psychiatric illness
   C. The length of the surgery
   D. The presence of soft neurological signs after surgery

Discussion

The patient is probably evidencing a postoperative organic brain syndrome, which is probably related to either an electrolyte imbalance, the stresses of surgery, blood loss, or brain damage perhaps related to hypoxia, which may have occurred during surgery. Alternately, the symptoms may be related to drug withdrawal or to drugs used during surgery. The chance of developing an organic brain syndrome after surgery increases with age, and is probably higher in patients with a prior history of psychiatric illness. In addition, the length of time in surgery and the presence of soft neurological signs developing after surgery increase the chances that an organic brain syndrome will be seen.

3. Treatment should include the following:
   A. The light should be shut off at night so that the patient can get adequate rest
   B. The patient should be kept in a room without windows, since it is likely he will jump out if he can
   C. Minor tranquilizers should be started, so that the patient gets adequate rest
   D. Relatives should be encouraged to visit the patient

Discussion

In handling patients with this confusional disorder, good nursing care is important: a calm, sympathetic, reassuring approach can turn a frightened patient into a cooperative one. Becuse such patients often misinterpret stimuli, it is important to provide a familiar, stable, and unambiguous environment for them. Simple, repeated explanations and frequent reassurances from familiar persons can be helpful. Patients do better with some light on at night and reminders of the time of day and day of the week. Patients also do better if familiar people, such as close relatives, are near. Sedatives and other central-nervous-system depressants are contraindicated, for they tend to increase the patient's confusion and excitement.

4. In selecting the correct drug for treating this patient, you are guided by which of the following general principles?
   A. It is best to avoid using medications in patients with an acute organic brain syndrome
   B. If a medication is used, the one with the lowest chances of producing hypotension should be used
   C. When drugs are used, one should use the smallest dose possible and increase the dose slowly
   D. If drugs are used, the ones with the lowest chance of giving parkinsonian side effects should be used

Discussion

Antipsychotic drugs can be a valuable adjunct in relieving symptoms of anxiety, impulsivity, depression, and paranoid ideation. They should be instituted quite carefully, however, and avoided if possible. If the patient does require chemical intervention, the drug instituted should be chosen as carefully for its side effects as for its primary actions. Only the smallest effective doses of drugs should be used, because organic-brain-syndrome patients are frequently very sensitive to these agents. No drug is entirely safe. Careful attention to dosage and mental status are more important than the particular drug used. In general, drugs that cause large drops in blood pressure should be avoided.

5. Characteristics of the patient with organic brain syndrome who needs medications include:
   A. The patient disrupts the general ward
   B. The patient's organicity is interfering with his medical workup
   C. Neurological and vital signs have been stable

Discussion

The usual indications for the use of antipsychotic drugs in confused patients are disturbance to the ward that is so great that it requires some form of restraint, and patients whose organicity is interfering with the ability of their physician to carry out an adequate medical workup due to lack of cooperation. In general, only patients who have stable vital signs should be given psychotropic medications.

Answers

1. (A and C)
2. (A, B, C, and D)
3. (D)
4. (A, B, and C)
5. (A, B, and C)

References

1. Barnes, R. F., Veith, R. C., Okimoto, J., Raskind, M., and Gumbrecht, G.: Efficacy of antipsychotic medications in behaviorally disturbed dementia patients. *American Journal of Psychiatry*, 139: 1170–1174, 1982.
2. Ray, W. A., Federspiel, C. F., and Schaffner, W.: A study of antipsychotic drug use in nursing homes: Epidemiologic evidence suggesting misuse. *American Journal of Public Health*, 70: 485–491, 1980.
3. Flaherty, J. A.: Psychiatric complications of medical drugs. *Journal of Family Practice*, 9(2): 243–251, 1979.
4. Danielson, D. A., Porter, J.B., Lawson, D. H., Soubrie, C., and Jick, H.: Drug-associated psychiatric disturbances in medical inpatients. *Psychopharmacology*, 74: 105–108, 1981.

CASE 46: CONFUSION IN AN ELDERLY MAN

A 74-year-old white man is admitted to the hospital after falling and fracturing his hip. On admission, he is moderately anxious, yet oriented and alert. Twenty-four hours after entering the hospital he becomes confused and disoriented to place and time. He mistakes people for others, see strange forms in the corner of his room, is afraid of being poisoned, and picks at his bedsheets. His temperature is 99°F. A physical examination is normal. During his stay in the hospital, he receives pentazocine (Talwin) for pain and chlordiazepoxide (Librium) for anxiety.

1. The differential diagnosis of this patient's confusional state should include:
   A. Talwin toxicity
   B. Disinhibition and confusion secondary to chlordiazepoxide
   C. Withdrawal from alcohol
   D. Withdrawal from sedative–hypnotics
   E. All of the above
   F. None of the above
2. Disinhibition and confusion in the elderly following clinical doses of chlordiazepoxide or diazepam (Valium):
   A. Are very rare
   B. Are relatively common
   C. Occur in virtually 100% of cases
   D. Never occur
3. The clinical course in the case of this patient would suggest alcohol or sedative–hypnotic withdrawal:
   A. Not at all
   B. Somewhat
   C. Moderately
   D. Certainly
4. Physical causes of the patient's development of confusion probably do not include:
   A. Senility
   B. Subdural hematoma
   C. Pneumonia

D. Cerebrovascular insufficiency
E. Pain syndrome

Discussion

The determination of the etiology of confusion in a previously mentally clear hospitalized patient is often difficult and frustrating. Such deterioration may be considered "a manifestation of senility," when the true etiology is actually traumatic, metabolic, or due to drug withdrawal. Development of confusion in an elderly patient should alert the physician to the possibility of central-nervous-system trauma such as subdural hematomas, systemic illnesses such as pneumonia or electrolyte imbalances, alcohol or sedative–hypnotic withdrawal, or psychotropic–drug toxicity. Virtually all narcotics or narcotic agonists can cause confusion, as can the minor tranquilizers such as chlordiazepoxide (Librium) or diazepam (Valium). Such effects are especially prevalent in the elderly. Thus, drugs with psychotropic effects are best used carefully in the treatment of the elderly, beginning with lower doses. Use of an antipsychotic agent such as haloperidol (Haldol) is probably preferable to diazepam or chlordiazepoxide in the treatment of psychotic elderly patients.

Answers

1. (E)
2. (B)
3. (C)
4. (A and E)

References

1. Caine, E.: Pseudodementia. *Archives in General Psychiatry*, 38: 1359, 1981.

SECTION V
DRUG AND ALCOHOL ABUSE

CASE 47: DIAZEPAM (VALIUM) DEPENDENCE

A 45-year-old, lonely, mildly anxious housewife has been using diazepam (Valium) for 2½ years. She takes six to eight 10-mg diazepam tablets per day. She has decided to stop her diazepam and join a religious cult. She plans to do this abruptly and mentions this while having a routine physical examination.

1. The patient:
   A. Can safely stop her diazepam
   B. Needs to taper her diazepam dose over a 2-week period
   C. Needs to continue her diazepam indefinitely
2. Diazepam may cause:
   A. Addiction
   B. Habituation
   C. Neither addiction or habituation
   D. Both addiction and habituation
3. The minimal intake of diazepam necessary to cause physical addiction is:
   A. 10 mg per day for 2 months or more
   B. 60 mg per day or more for 1½ months or more
   C. 100 mg per day or more for 4 or more months
   D. 100 mg per day for 1 week

Discussion

Diazepam is a moderately addicting drug. If a patient has been using this drug for 1½ or more months, in doses greater than 60 mg per day, withdrawal symptoms with drug cessation are likely. Diazepam can also cause habituation. Patients who have been taking relatively high doses of this drug are best advised to taper their dose slowly, over a period of weeks. Withdrawal from diazepam can present as anxiety and agitation, or be severe and manifested as seizures, delirium, and vasomotor instability.

Case Continued: The patient attends the religious meeting and is informed that she isn't sincere enough to be a part of the cult. She returns home and overdoses on her diazepam. She ingests 60 mg. She then calls her gynecologist.

4. It is likely that:
   A. The patient will die before she reaches the hospital
   B. The patient will become psychotic
   C. The patient will survive
5. Diazepam-induced central nervous system depression is more likely to occur in:
   A. Elderly persons
   B. Patients with low serum albumin levels
   C. All of the above
   D. None of the above

Discussion

Diazepam is a relatively safe drug in an overdose. The lethal dose in animals is very high. Therefore, although lavage, supportive care, and other measures are indicated following an overdose, the chances of death are minimal. However, it is likely that diazepam in combination with sedative-hypnotics or alcohol enhances the rather severe toxicity of these agents in an overdose. It is preferable to use an antianxiety agent such as flurazepam (Dalmane) as a soporific, rather than a sedative-hypnotic. Metabolic characteristics of the patient will differentially determine the depressive effects on the central nervous system.

Answers

1. (B)
2. (D)
3. (B)
4. (C)
5. (C)

References

1. Greenblatt, D. J. and Shader, R. I.: I. Benzodiazepines. *New England Journal of Medicine*, 291: 1011–1015, 1974.
2. Greenblatt, D. J. and Shader, R. I.: II. Benztropines. *New England Journal of Medicine*, 291: 1239–1243, 1974.
3. Hall, R. C. W. and Jaffe, J. R.: Aberrant response to diazepam: A new syndrome. *American Journal of Psychiatry*, 129: 738–742, 1972.
4. Boston Collaborative Drug Surveillance Program: Clinical depression of the central nervous system due to diazepam and chlordiazepoxide in relation to cigarette smoking and age. *New England Journal of Medicine*, 288: 277–280. 1973.
5. Shader, R. I. and Greenblatt, D. J.: Clinical implications of benzodiazepines: Pharmacokinetics. *American Journal of Psychiatry*, 134(6): 652–656, 1977.

CASE 48: SEDATIVE-HYPNOTIC OVERDOSE

A 37-year-old white woman has been separated from her husband for 8 months. She is brought to the emergency room after a call by her children to a neighbor. They returned from school and found their mother lying in the bedroom in an unresponsive state. A bottle of 100-mg pentobarbital tablets was found at her side. On admission to the emergency room she is unresponsive to verbal stimuli. She appears dizzy, severely ataxic, confused, and has barely audible, slurred speech. The neighbor relates that she has had an increasingly difficult time adjusting since she has been separated from her husband, and she has used barbiturates on a regular basis in order to deal with her grief. She has recently been talking of feeling that life was not worth living if the marriage could not be reconciled. The patient, in addition, has been drinking alcohol, and there is a distinct alcohol odor on her breath.

1. Usually, severe intoxication will be produced by ingestion of pentobarbital in a dose of:
   A. 100 to 200 mg
   B. 200 to 1,000 mg
   C. 600 to 1,500 mg
   D. 1,000 to 1,500 mg
   E. 2,000 to 4,000 mg

Discussion

Severe sedative–hypnotic intoxication is produced by the acute ingestion of 200 to 1,000 mg pentobarbital. The fatal dose is only slightly higher, being around 1,000 to 1,500 mg.

2. The additional use of alcohol in this patient would:
   A. Have no effect
   B. Have an additive or synergistic effect
   C. Sedate, but not contribute to the effect of pentobarbital
   D. Stimulate the patient's metabolism of pentobarbital, therefore diminishing its potentially lethal effect
   E. Only make the patient uncooperative
   F. Make one suspect gastrointestinal disease because of its effects

Discussion

As little as eight tablets of pentobarbital 100 mg when taken with alcohol, can result in death. Thus, alcohol and the barbiturates may have an additive, or possibly a synergistic effect.

3. Appropriate treatment of this patient would include:
   A. Ipecac 300 cc p.o., STAT
   B. Gastric lavage
   C. Intravenous fluids
   D. All of the above

Discussion

The emptying of the patient's stomach by inducing vomiting, if the patient is conscious, or by lavage if the patient is unconscious, is of extreme importance in treating a sedative–hypnotic overdose, since this prevents further absorption of the drug. Lavage or induced vomiting is useful even several hours after the drug has been ingested, since some drugs are absorbed slowly from the gastrointestinal tract. However, vomiting should not be induced in the unconscious patient because of the danger of aspiration. Continuous nursing care, based on anesthesiologic principles, is essential in the treatment of sedative–hypnotic overdose, especially in the presence of respiratory depression. Endotracheal intubation and external respiratory support may be required.

4. Sixteen hours after the institution of emergency care the patient's sensorium is clear. The possibility that a significant barbiturate withdrawal syndrome may develop is present if the patient has been on barbiturates (or sedative–hypnotics) continually for a:
   A. 2-week period
   B. 1-month period
   C. 3-month period
   D. 6-month period

Discussion

Barbiturate addiction develops only when approximately 400 to 600 mg of pentobarbital or an equivalent dose of another sedative–hypnotic is taken daily for a period of 1½ to 3 months. Tolerance to barbiturate toxicity does not occur. Thus, the addict may become resistant to the hypnotic effects of sedative–hypnotics without the lethal dose being significantly increased.

5. In untreated cases, a barbiturate-withdrawal syndrome tends to subside in approximately:
   A. 3 days
   B. 8 days
   C. 21 days

Discussion

The withdrawal syndrome that follows the use of large amounts of sedative hypnotics, taken over extended periods, ususally subsides spontaneously in approximately 8 days.

6. Signs and symptoms expected to occur with 36 hours following the last dose of a chronically ingested barbiturate include which of the following?
   A. Restlessness and anxiety
   B. Tremulousness and weakness
   C. Seizures
   D. Abdominal cramps and nausea
   E. Orthostatic hypotension
   F. All of the above

Discussion

Twelve to 48 hours after withdrawal from chronic barbiturate ingestion, the patient may show weakness, tremor, anxiety, and restlessness, as well as orthostatic hypotension. Nausea, abdominal cramps, and vomiting may occur. Seizures may not occur until 72 hours following the last dose of a barbiturate. This can be especially important in the patient who appears improved in all other parameters, but then develops a seizure. Associated symptoms during withdrawal also frequently include a clouded sensorium, disorientation, severe agitation, and in some cases hypothermia.

7. In order to prevent withdrawal seizures, a specific program of detoxification can be decided upon by:
   A. Obtaining a careful history from the patient
   B. Dividing the patient's admitted sedative–hypnotic dose in half
   C. Giving a test dose of 200 mg of pentobarbital
   D. Maintenance on diazepam will suffice
   E. None of the above

Case Continued: You decide to gradually withdraw the patient from barbiturates over a period of 7 to 10 days. Your starting daily dose of pentobarbital (a short-acting barbiturate) is to be decided by giving a test dose of pentobarbital 200 mg p.o. In the following four questions, match the expected daily dose of pentobarbital required for successful withdrawal with symptoms seen 1 hour after a test dose of pentobarbital 200 mg p.o. has been given.

8. No sign of drug effect in 1 hour:
   A. Pentobarbital 0 mg per day
   B. Pentobarbital 400 to 600 mg per day
   C. Pentobarbital 800 mg per day
   D. Pentobarbital 1,000 to 1,200 mg per day
   E. Unlikely to have physical dependency
9. Fine lateral gaze nystagmus only:
   A. Pentobarbital 0 mg per day
   B. Pentobarbital 400 to 600 mg per day
   C. Pentobarbital 800 mg per day
   D. Pentobarbital 1,000 to 1,200 mg per day
   E. Unlikely to have physical dependency
10. Drowsy and ataxic with slurred speech:
    A. Pentobarbital 0 mg per day
    B. Pentobarbital 400 to 600 mg per day
    C. Pentobarbital 800 mg per day
    D. Pentobarbital 1,000 to 1,200 mg per day
    E. Unlikely to have physical dependency
11. Asleep:
    A. Pentobarbital 0 to 100 mg per day
    B. Pentobarbital 400 to 600 mg per day
    C. Pentobarbital 800 mg per day
    D. Pentobarbital 1,000 to 1,200 mg per day
    E. Unlikely to have physical dependency

Discussion

If the patient is found to be asleep, but arousable after a 200-mg test dose of pentobarbital, the degree of tolerance is usually negligible, and the patient is not a sedative–hypnotic addict. If the patient is found to be drowsy and ataxic, with slurred speech and coarse lateral gaze nystagmus, a tolerance can be presumed to exist and a daily 500-to 600-mg barbiturate (pentobarbital) requirement per 24 hours probably exists. If the patient is found to appear normal, having only fine lateral nystagmus, a moderate tolerance probably exists and a pentobarbital requirement of 800 mg per day may be assumed. If there is no sign of a drug effect following 200 mg pentobarbital, and, the patient shows continued restlessness, an extreme tolerance exists, and a dose of 1,000 to 1,200 mg or more per day of pentobarbital may be presumed to be the patient's daily barbiturate requirement. However, it is important to note that the above test is relatively crude. It is best to use the pentobarbital test dose to reach a general dosage, and then dose range up or down, depending on the patient's responses. Pentobarbital should be given every 4 to 6 hours in doses that keep the patient intoxicated (dysarthric, ataxic, etc.) for at least 24 hours before withdrawal is begun. Such a technique prevents too rapid a lowering of the barbiturate dose.

12. After the intoxicating dose of barbiturate has been established, the barbiturate (pentobarbital or secobarbital) is usually withdrawn at the rate of:
    A. 5% of the total daily dose or less per day
    B. 10% of the total daily dose or less per day
    C. 50% of the total daily dose per day
    D. 75% of the total daily dose per day

Discussion

Barbiturate reduction should not exceed 100 mg per day, which is usually 10% or less of the total daily stabilizing dose. If the patient shows increasing symptoms of abstinence during the withdrawal, the withdrawal rate should be slowed, extra doses of barbituate should be given, or both.

13. The average period usually necessary for withdrawal from chronic barbiturate or sedative–hypnotic ingestion is:
    A. 2 to 4 days
    B. 5 to 10 days
    C. 10 to 21 days
    D. 18 to 30 days

Discussion

Withdrawal from barbiturates or other sedative–hypnotics usually can be completed within 10 to 21 days. Useful adjunctive medication during the withdrawal may include sodium diphenylhydantoin (Dilantin). Dilantin may be indicated in patients who have had a history of seizures in the past, either as a result of sedative–hypnotic or alcohol withdrawal, or from other causes.

14. Following detoxification, symptoms experienced by the patient may include:
    A. Hypersomnolence and apathy
    B. Insomnia and irritability
    C. Neither
    D. Both

Discussion

Before discharge, it is essential to tell the patient that he or she may have some insomnia and irritability for several more weeks or even months. It is believed that these symptoms are based on physiological factors, although emotional components cannot be discounted.

Answers

1. (B)
2. (B)
3. (D)
4. (C)
5. (B)
6. (F)
7. (A and C)
8. (D)
9. (C)
10. (B)
11. (A)
12. (B)
13. (C)
14. (D)

References

1. Ewing, J. A. and Bakewell, W. E.: Diagnosis and management of depressive drug dependence. *American Journal of Psychiatry*, 123: 909–917, 1967.

2. Oswald, I. and Priest, R. G.: Five weeks to escape the sleeping pill habit. *British Journal of Medicine*, 2: 1093–1095, 1965.

CASE 49: DRUG TREATMENT OF THE ALCOHOLIC

A 40-year-old postal worker is brought to the emergency room by his wife because of a tremor of rapid onset and general anxiety. The patient has been a heavy drinker for many years, and has increased his intake to a pint of whiskey daily over the past 2 months. The psychiatric history is otherwise negative, and you diagnosis impending alcoholic withdrawal and begin treatment.

1. Good general rules to follow in treating withdrawal include the following:
   A. A thorough physical examination is mandatory
   B. Treatment of overhydration may be necessary
   C. A subdural hematoma must be carefully ruled out
   D. As a rule, alcoholic withdrawal should occur in a hospital
2. Correct statements about the drug treatment of alcoholic withdrawal include:
   A. Almost any depressant drug can be used
   B. Paraldehyde offers the advantage of being easily administered, both orally and intramuscularly
   C. Chlordiazepoxide (Librium) offers the advantage of causing only mild changes in blood pressure
   D. Care should be taken to not use intoxicating levels of the depressant drugs

Discussion

As a general rule, alcoholic withdrawal should occur in a hospital. An essential part of the treatment is a thorough physical examination, along with chest and skull films to rule out medical problems such as pneumonia, heart failure, and subdural hematomas, which may have precipitated the withdrawal or occur with it. Blood tests should be used to evaluate the presence of pancreatitis, infection, and the degree of hydration. It has recently been established that most alcoholics in withdrawal are overhydrated. A number of diuretics, including furosemide (80 mg every 3 hours p.o.) have been recommended, but the fluid balance of each patient should be individually evaluated. One approach to treating alcoholic withdrawal is to give enough of a depressant drug that has a cross-tolerance with alcohol to control withdrawal symptoms, and then decrease the dose of this drug slowly. Almost any depressant drug can be used, and the specific medication chosen is often dependent on the side effects one wishes to avoid, and one's clinical experience. Paraldehyde has frequently been used, but offers the disadvantage of being neurotoxic if injected too close to a nerve. Chlordiazepoxide offers the advantages of oral and parental administration and of causing only mild postural hypotension.

3. You choose to use chlordiazepoxide. Correct statements about its use include:
   A. This drug effectively controls withdrawal seizures
   B. The drug should be continued for a minimum of 12 months before it is stopped
   C. Proper use of this drug in the early stages of withdrawal will probably avoid full-blown delirium tremens

Discussion

The rationale for the use of chlordiazepoxide is that physiologic addiction can be alleviated by slowly decreasing the level of the addicting drug or a drug with a cross-tolerance to it. The initial dose of chlordiazepoxide needs to be individually titrated, but most alcoholics require 200 to 400 mg per day given orally or intravenously, in divided 50- to 100-mg doses every 3 to 4 hours. Final doses thus range from 200 to 500 mg on the first day, and the drug is then decreased by about 20% per day. Controlled studies indicate that chlordiazepoxide works well in the treatment of alcohol withdrawal, decreasing the incidence of organic brain syndrome and withdrawal seizures. Due to the addictive potential of this drug, however, the medication should be stopped when withdrawal is complete, usually 5 days to a week after beginning treatment.

4. Your treatment of withdrawal is likely to include:
   A. Diphenylhydantoin (Dilantin) for controlling drug-induced seizures

B. Thiamine in doses of 100 mg i.m. daily for at least the first week
C. Megavitamin therapy

Discussion

Diphenylhydantoin has been tried in the treatment of alcohol withdrawal. While this drug is usually added in an attempt to control withdrawal seizures, its use is based on impressions from uncontrolled trials. There is no firm evidence that diphenylhydantoin works in controlling withdrawal seizures, or that it is essential for permitting alcoholic withdrawal if other depressants are properly administered. Essential in the proper treatment of the alcoholic is the addition of thamine in doses of 100 mg intramuscularly for at least the first week, and the use of multiple vitamins. There is no good evidence that megavitamin dosage is additionally effective.

5. In evaluating the progress of the withdrawal, one should be aware that:
   A. The withdrawal may begin while the patient still has a relatively high blood-alcohol level
   B. The withdrawal is likely to peak in intensity after 2 or 3 days
   C. The withdrawal will probably be complete by 5 or 6 days
   D. The use of drugs in the treatment of withdrawal does nothing to modify the mortality rate of the withdrawal process

Discussion

The alcoholic withdrawal syndrome is typical of the depressant-abstinence syndromes. It is characterized by anxiety, involuntary twitching, a coarse tremor, progressive weakness, and dizziness. These symptoms may progress to autonomic nervous system dysfunction, convulsions, an agitated confusion or delirium, and hallucinations—usually tactile and visual. The symptoms can begin within 4 to 12 hours after the alcohol intake has been decreased (not that the blood-alcohol level does not necessarily have to be zero). The symptoms reach their maximum intensity on the second or third day, and then decline over the next 2 to 5 days. If treated properly, with good medical care, the alcohol-withdrawal syndrome rarely becomes a full-blown delirium tremens (tremors, delirium, autonomic nervous system dysfunction, and visual hallucinations), and the mortality rate is relatively low.

Case Continued: The patient described in this case was successfully withdrawn from alcohol. You are then asked by the patient, as well as his family, to institute rehabilitative care.

6. You consider using disulfiram (Antabuse). Correct statements about the use of this drug include:
   A. Patients with hypertension, cirrhosis, or cardiac disease should not be treated with this drug
   B. Its major action is the blockade of alcohol dehydrogenase
   C. The disulfiram reaction usually occurs within 15 minutes of the ingestion of alcohol
   D. The death rate from the alcohol–disulfiram reaction is approximately 2%

Discussion

Disulfiram acts by blocking aldehyde dehydrogenase, so that toxic levels of acetaldehyde develop within minutes after alcohol is consumed. The alcohol–disulfiram interaction begins with facial flushing, followed by headache and hypertension, which gives way to precipitous hypotension, faintness, nausea, and vomiting, lasting up to 1 hour. One-half of a 500-mg tablet of disulfiram is given daily, with the result that the patient cannot drink alcohol without suffering a severe reaction. The drug has not been shown to curb the drive to drink. Disulfiram alone is associated with a low level of adverse effects, but its reaction with alcohol can be fatal, although it rarely is (much less than 1%). Patients with serious cardiovascular difficulties or other major health problems should be excluded from treatment with disulfiram.

7. You consider using minor tranquilizers. Correct statements about the use of these drugs in the treatment of alcoholic rehabilitation include:
   A. The intoxication from these drugs is clinically similar to the intoxication from alcohol

B. These drugs can be physiologically addicting
C. It has been found that these drugs may increase pre-existing depression, and thus raise the patient's suicide potential
D. These drugs have consistently been shown to be better than placebo in alleviating the chronic anxiety that drives alcoholics to drink

Discussion

Minor tranquilizers are frequently used as adjuncts to other therapies in an attempt to decrease the alcoholic's level of anxiety, on the assumption that higher anxiety levels lead to and maintain alcoholism. Minor tranquilizers, however, may themselves be physically addictive. Their similarity to alcohol may make it difficult for alcoholics to control their intake, and there are also reports that minor tranquilizers may increase the level of pre-existing depression or raise the patient's suicide potential. In addition, these drugs have not been shown to be effective in the treatment of chronic anxiety, and thus their long-term use in the treatment of alcoholism does not seem particularly indicated.

8. The patient complains of sadness and some despair regarding the future. You consider using antidepressants. Correct statements about these drugs and the treatment of alcoholism include:
   A. In alcoholics, the symptom of sadness does not necessarily indicate the presence of an affective disorder
   B. In alcoholics, the depressive affect tends to lift after withdrawal
   C. The dangers of mixing tricyclic antidepressants and alcohol suggest that these antidepressants should be prescribed only with extreme care in alcoholism
   D. Repeated controlled studies have shown lithium to be better than placebo in the treatment of alcoholism

Discussion

A number of medications have been advocated for use in the treatment of alcoholic rehabilitation. One must be careful not to confuse a report of a depressive mood with the diagnosis of major depressive disorder; thus, not all alcoholics complaining of depression require antidepressant medication. The efficacy of lithium or tricyclic antidepressant medications for alcoholics has not been tested in well-controlled studies. Most studies in which antidepressants have been used routinely for alcoholics give favorable results, but these are only uncontrolled reports. Controlled studies, on the other hand, indicate no superiority for tricyclics or monoamine oxidase inhibitors over minor tranquilizers or placebos. There is also an additional danger since antidepressants and lithium may have adverse interactions with alcohol.

9. Correct statements about the use of the following drugs in alcoholic rehabilitation include:
   A. Controlled studies have not shown lysergic acid diethylamide to be effective in the long-term treatment of alcoholism
   B. Metronidazole (Flagyl) has been shown in controlled studies to have both disulfiram-like properties and to cut down on the drive of the alcoholic to drink
   C. In general, all drugs look effective in uncontrolled alcoholic rehabilitation studies
   D. Amphetamines have been shown in controlled studies to be effective in the long-term management of the depression sometimes associated with alcoholism

Discussion

Because of the high rate of spontaneous remission in alcoholism, almost any drug used in uncontrolled studies appears effective. Because of this, drugs such as metronidazole and lysergic acid diethylamide (LSD) have been used in alcoholic rehabilitation and found to be effective, but only in uncontrolled trials. As these drugs are exposed to controlled evaluation, claims of their effectiveness disappear. Another example of this phenomenon occurs with stimulants, which have been used to deal with the depression and lack of energy that may follow alcohol withdrawal. Here, no controlled studies have been done, and a potentially high risk of abuse for these drugs makes them ill suited for clinical use in alcoholics.

Answers

1. (A, B, C, and D)
2. (A and C)
3. (A and C)
4. (B)
5. (A, B, and C)
6. (A and C)
7. (A, B, and C)
8. (A, B, and C)
9. (A and C)

References

1. Palestine, M. L.: Drug treatment of the alcohol withdrawal syndrome and delerium tremens. *Quarterly Journal of Studies on Alcohol*, 34: 185–193, 1973.
2. Knott, D. H. and Beard, J. D.: The diuretic approach to acute withdrawal from alcohol. *Southern Medical Journal*, 62: 485–488, 1969.
3. Greenblatt, D. J. and Shader, R. I.: *Benzodiazepines in Clinical Practice.* Raven Press, New York, 1974.
4. Kiam, S. C., Klett, C. J., and Rothfeld, B.: Treatment of the acute withdrawal state: A comparison of four drugs. *American Journal of Psychiatry*, 24: 174–178, 1971.
5. Adams, H. P.: Diphenylhydantoin in the treatment of alcohol withdrawal. *Journal of the American Medical Association*, 218: 598, 1971.
6. Gessner, P. E.: Is diphenylhydantoin effective in the treatment of alcoholic withdrawal? *Journal of the American Medical Association*, 219: 1072, 1972.
7. Detre, T. P. and Jarecki, H. G.: *Modern Psychiatric Treatment*. J. B. Lippincott Co., Philadelphia, 1970, pp. 221–226.
8. Etzioni, A. and Remp, R.: *Technological Shortcuts to Social Change*. Russell Sage Foundation, New York, 1973, p. 53.
9. Schuckit, M. A.: Depression and alcoholism in women. In: *Proceedings of the First Annual Conference of the National Institute of Alcohol Abuse and Alcoholism: Research on Alcoholism: Clinical Problems and Special Populations*. National Institute of Mental Health, Bethesda, MD, 1973.
10. Overall, J. E., Brown, D., and Williams, J. D.: Drug treatment of anxiety and depression in detoxified alcoholic patients. *Archives of General Psychiatry*, 29: 218–221, 1973.
11. Schuckit, M. A. and Cahalan, D.: Evaluation of alcohol treatment programs. In: *Drugs in Combination with Other Therapies* (ed.: M. Greenblatt). Grune and Stratton, New York, 1975.
12. Shader, R. I.: *Psychiatric Complications of Medical Drugs*. Raven Press, New York, 1972, pp. 175–199.

13. Schattler, E. K. E. and Lal, S.: Treatment of alcoholism with Dent's oral apomorphine method. *Quarterly Journal of Studies on Alcohol*, 33: 430–436, 1972.
14. Bandura, A. L.: *Principles of Behavior Modification*. Holt, Rinehart and Winston, New York, 1969, pp. 538–551.
15. Gorelick, D. A.: Pharmacotherapy of alcohol and drug abuse. *Psychiatric Annals*, 13(1): 71–79, 1983.
16. Sellers, E. M. and Kacant, H.: Alcohol intoxication and withdrawal. *New England Journal of Medicine*, 294: 757–762, 1976.

CASE 50: WITHDRAWAL FROM DIAZEPAM

A 63-year-old widowed white woman presents for treatment of her chronic depression at a psychiatric mental-health clinic. She gives a 25-year history of having been chronically depressed and feeling hopeless, being insomniac (stating that she hasn't had a good night's sleep in 15 years), and having never been able to enjoy life. She claims to feel no sex drive. She reports frequent frontal headaches and backaches of 30 years duration. A mental-status examination shows the patient to be moderately sad-appearing. In reviewing the patient's medication history, she reports that she has been given a series of antidepressants and anti-anxiety agents over the past 20 years. Her past medications have included amitriptyline, imipramine, desipramine, trazodone, doxepin, diazepam, tenazepam, meprobanate, chlordiazepoxide, thyroid extract, gelusil, and propoxyphene.

For the past 6 months the patient has been taking desipramine 150 mg per day at bedtime, diazepam 10 mg, q.i.d. and 20 mg at bedtime, and propoxyphene, 64 mg, t.i.d. The patient is seen in the clinic by a psychiatric resident who decides that her diazepam probably is not helping her. He refills her propoxyphene and desipramine prescriptions, but tells the patient that he does not want to refill the diazepam because "it could addict you or cause side effects."

1. Given the length of diazepam treatment and the dosage given in this case, the risk of a withdrawal reaction is:
   A. Very low
   B. Moderate
   C. Nonexistent

2. Serious withdrawal reactions from benzodiazepines are most likely to occur because of:
   A. Prolonged usage
   B. Higher than recommended doses
   C. Abrupt discontinuation
   D. All of the above
   E. None of the above
3. Withdrawal from benzodiazepines is most likely to occur with prolonged treatment using:
   A. Short-acting agents
   B. Long-acting agents
   C. Intermediate-acting agents
   D. None of the above

Discussion

Although not usually as severe as with the barbiturates and sedative–hypnotics, a withdrawal syndrome can occur following the abrupt cessation of long-term, high-dose treatment with benzodiazepine derivatives. For example, withdrawal of diazepam 60 mg per day following treatment for 6 weeks can lead to a withdrawal reaction. Therefore, a withdrawal reaction in the case described above is likely. Since the long-acting benzodiazepine derivatives and their metabolites exit slowly from the blood stream, the risk of a withdrawal reaction is less likely than with a short-acting antianxiety agent. Furthermore, withdrawal reactions are more intense and occur earlier in patients taking short-acting benzodiazepine derivatives.

Case Continued: As could have been predicted, the patient returns for her next appointment 8 days after discontinuing diazepam and reports that she has become increasingly jittery, insomniac, anxious, and irritable over the past week. She reports that 2 days previously she visited her internist, who prescribed chlordiazepoxide 10 mg, q.i.d. for her nervousness, and that she now feels depressed but is sleeping better. She says she feels she would like to continue her chlordiazepoxide, since it has worked so well.

4. The side effects of benzodiazepines frequently include:
   A. Sedation
   B. Ataxia
   C. Hypotension
   D. Fainting
   E. A and B
   F. C and D
5. In patients who have been chronically using moderate doses of benzodiazepine derivatives:
   A. The drug must be withdrawn to avoid addiction
   B. It may often be necessary to continue the benzodiazepine as previously
   C. A slow decrease in dosage is indicated
   D. A and C
   E. B and C

Discussion

Very often, psychiatrists, and especially inexperienced ones, are overzealous in their efforts at preventing or stopping patients from taking the benzodiazepine antianxiety agents. Although such agents are overprescribed, and in general should be avoided except for short-term, low-dose usage, the reality is that these drugs are widely and chronically used by many people, and many patients are either habituated or addicted to them. Arbitrarily discontinuing such agents is not the treatment of choice. The clinician should be sensitive to the need to slowly wean such patients from their benzodiazepine, and in many cases such discontinuation may be essentially impossible. Such withdrawal, if it is to occur, should occur within the context of a consensual therapeutic relationship, with the patient agreeing about its desirability.

Answers

1. (B)
2. (D)
3. (A)
4. (E)
5. (E)

References

1. Gillin, J. C. and Mendelson, W. B.: Sleeping pills: For whom? When? How long? In: *Neuropharmacology of Central Nervous System and Behavioral Disorders* (ed.: G. C. Palmer). Academic Press, New York, 1981, pp. 285–316.
2. Kupfer, D. J., Spiker, D. G., Coble, P. A., *et al.*: Sleep and treatment prediction in endogenous depression. *American Journal of Psychiatry*, 138(4): 429–434, 1981.
3. Pitts, W. M., Fann, W. E., Sajadi, C., and Snyder, S.: Alprazolam in older depressed inpatients. *Journal of Clinical Psychiatry*, 44: 213–215, 1983.
4. Feighner, J. P.: Open label study of alprazolam in severely depressed inpatients. *Journal of Clinical Psychiatry*, 44: 332–334, 1983.
5. Salzman, C., Shader, R. I., Greenblatt, D. J., Horwatz, J. S., and Long, V. S.: Short half-life benzodiazepines in the elderly. *Archives of General Psychiatry*, 40: 293–297, 1983.
6. Greenblatt, D. J., Sellers, E. M., and Shader, R. I.: Drug disposition in old age. *New England Journal of Medicine*, 306: 1081–1088, 1982.
7. Greenblatt, D. J., Divall, M., Abernathy, D. R., *et al.*: Alprazolam kinetics in the elderly. *Archives of General Psychiatry*, 40: 287–290, 1983.

CASE 51: TREATMENT OF WERNICKE-KORSAKOFF SYNDROME

The patient is a 52-year-old white male for whom you are called to consult because of memory impairment. The patient entered the hospital approximately 2 weeks prior to your seeing him, in a state of alcoholic withdrawal. The withdrawal was treated properly, and within 5 days the patient's major symptoms had largely cleared, leaving him in a somewhat confused state. The confusion appeared to remit, but the patient then developed memory impairment, most marked for recent events. Your examination reveals a pleasant, cooperative man who appears to have an intact remote memory but grossly impaired recent memory. Otherwise, the mental-status examination is within normal limits.

1. Correct statements about the effect of alcohol on the central nervous system include:
   A. It probably has direct neurotoxic effects unrelated to vitamin deficiency

B. The frontal–parietal areas are frequently atrophic in chronic alcoholics
C. Enlarged ventricles are frequently seen in alcoholics with brain damage
D. One common gross pathologic finding in alcoholics is atrophy of the occipital lobes

2. Correct statements about Wernicke–Korsakoff syndrome include:
   A. Its onset is usually before age 35
   B. In the acute stages of the disorder, when the symptoms of Wernicke's and Korsakoff's syndromes appear at the same time, two-thirds of the patients show confusion
   C. The major contributing factor to this disorder is the toxic effect of alcohol
   D. In the acute phases, ocular palsies are seen in nearly one-half of the patients

Discussion

While the final answer is not clear, there is strong evidence that, in addition to vitamin deficiency and trauma as causes of central nervous system damage in alcoholics, alcohol itself probably has a direct neurotoxic effect. No matter what the cause is, cortical atrophy occurs in alcoholics (most marked in the frontal and parietal areas), along with enlargement of the cerebral ventricles. Wernicke's encephalopathy is an acute disorder, characterized by nystagmus and other ocular abnormalities, along with ataxia and mental confusion. It occurs most frequently in men aged 40 to 55, and it is a direct result of thiamine deficiency. The symptoms of Wernicke's and Korsakoff's syndromes are frequently combined, with the following symptoms being predominant: confusion in two-thirds of the patients, staggering in one-half, ocular palsies in one-half, polyneuropathy in almost 40%, laboratory findings of anemia in 40%, elevated liver function tests in almost one-half and EEG abnormalities in approximately one-half.

3. Correct statements about the treatment of Wernicke's syndrome include:
   A. Sixth-nerve palsy is a frequently observed finding which often improves within 24 hours with thiamine treatment

B. Less than half of patients with ataxia recover completely
C. Complete recovery can be seen with thiamine (50 to 100 mg daily)
D. The death rate in Wernicke's syndrome is about 25%

Discussion

In Wernicke's syndrome, a sixth-nerve palsy is the most frequent cranial-nerve finding. This responds to treatment with 50 to 100 mg of thiamine, injected daily, with great improvement frequently seen within 24 hours. Ataxia is much less likely to remit, with a final recovery rate of less than 40%. A global confusional state characterized by drowsiness, inattentiveness, disorientation, illusions, and misidentification frequently accompanies Wernicke–Korsakoff syndrome. With treatment, improvement occurs within about 2 weeks in most patients. The overall death rate for Wernicke–Korsakoff patients is quite low.

4. Correct statements about the course and diagnosis of Korsakoff's syndrome include:
   A. The diagnosis is based on observing markedly impaired memory functions, associated with an otherwise clear sensorium
   B. Approximately 25% of patients with Korsakoff's syndrome never recover, even partially
   C. Approximately 20% of patients with Korsakoff's syndrome recover completely
   D. Prompt use of thiamine prevents progression of the disease and reverses some of the lesions completely
5. The proper treatment of Korsakoff's syndrome includes:
   A. Thiamine 100 mg per day
   B. Strict bed rest
   C. A balanced diet and administration of all B vitamins, in addition to thiamine
   D. The use of minor tranquilizers in doses similar to those used for the treatment of alcoholic withdrawal

Discussion

Korsakoff's syndrome is diagnosed by the presence of a markedly impaired memory associated with an otherwise clear sensorium. The diagnosis carries a relatively poor prognosis, with over one-quarter of patients with the syndrome never recovering and only one-fifth recovering completely. Thiamine is the best treatment for this disorder. It prevents symptom progression and can reverse neurological deficiencies or lesions. In treating the disorder, it is advisable to use bed rest and keep a close watch for the development of congestive heart failure (associated with malnutrition). Treatment should also include a balanced diet, including all of the B vitamins. The onset of the memory loss in Korsakoff's psychosis may be delayed for several weeks or months after alcohol withdrawal. Recovery is unpredictable and may take months.

Answers

1. (A, B, and C)
2. (B and D)
3. (A, B, and C)
4. (A, B, C, and D)
5. (A, B, and C)

References

1. Parsons, O. A.: Brain damage in alcoholics: Altered states of unconsciousness. In: *Second Biannual International Symposium on Experimental Studies of Alcohol Interaction and Withdrawal* (ed.: M. Gross). Plenum Press, New York, 1975.
2. Hoffman, F. G.: *A Handbook on Drug and Alcohol Abuse.* Oxford University Press, New York, 1975, pp. 101–116.
3. Victor, M., Adams, R. D., and Collins, G. H.: *The Wernicke–Korsakoff Syndrome.* F. A. Davis Co., Philadelphia, 1971.

CASE 52: HEROIN DETOXIFICATION IN A YOUNG WOMAN

A 22-year-old white female college graduate is admitted to a medical unit for detoxification from heroin. She claims that she has a $350-per-day heroin habit and has been using heroin daily for 2 years. She now wishes to stop using this drug, stating that her habit is too expensive and that she wishes to "be clean." She states that her last "fix" (injection of heroin) was 2½ hours previously. The patient is physically healthy, without any serious abnormalities.

1. Abrupt withdrawal of the patient's heroin will invariably lead to:
   A. Serious toxicity and possibly death
   B. Seizures
   C. Uncomfortable but relatively safe withdrawal symptoms
   D. No physical sequelae
2. It is elected to treat the patient pharmacologically. The following drugs are indicated in heroin detoxification:
   A. Secobarbital (Seconal)
   B. Doxepin (Sinequan)
   C. Methadone
   D. Chlordiazepoxide (Librium)
   E. Atropine
   F. Clonidine
   G. All of the above
3. A reasonable starting dose of methadone is:
   A. 150 mg per day
   B. 100 mg per day
   C. 40 mg per day
   D. 5 mg per day
4. The methadone should be tapered over a:
   A. 20-day period
   B. 10-day period
   C. 6-day period
   D. 2-day period

Discussion

Abrupt withdrawal of heroin is not dangerous in a healthy individual. It is, however, an uncomfortable experience. Thus, "cold-turkey" withdrawal is a reasonable treatment procedure from a medical point of view. However, heroin withdrawal does lead to many cholinergic side effects which are quite uncomfortable and painful. Use of an antianxiety agent, a tricyclic antidepressant, and an anticholinergic agent may help decrease the above withdrawal effects. Traditionally, methadone is used to detoxify heroin addicts. A starting dose of methadone of 30 to 50 mg per day is acceptable, and this should be decreased to zero over a 6- to 8-day period. The doses are often given on a b.i.d. or t.i.d. basis. Propoxyphene napsylate (Darvon-N) has received widespread attention as a withdrawal agent, since it has considerable cross-tolerance with the opiates. Since propoxyphene napsylate is not recognized as a specific treatment for narcotic dependence by the U. S. Food and Drug Administration, however, its use as such is only investigative. Clonidine has recently been shown to abort narcotic-withdrawal symptoms, and does not itself cause withdrawal symptoms.

Case Continued: The patient is begun on a methadone detoxification program. She is started on 50 mg per day of methadone. It is planned that this be decreased over a 6-day period. On the second day of methadone withdrawal, the patient receives 40 mg. She begins to complain that she is experiencing cramping, sweating, and anxiety. She begs for more methadone and says she needs a slower detoxification schedule.

5. The appropriate course of action is to:
   A. Increase the methadone dosage to 85 mg per day
   B. Continue on the designated program, reassure the patient, and offer an anticholinergic drug, an antianxiety drug, or both as needed.
   C. Tell the patient to stop faking her symptoms since she physically cannot be having withdrawal
6. An alternate course of action would be to:
   A. Use insulin-coma therapy
   B. Allow the patient to detoxify herself, giving her a specific number of methadone tablets to utilize over a specific period
   C. Discharge the patient for being manipulative
   D. Inject naloxone (Narcan)
   E. Use clonidine to alleviate the patient's withdrawal symptoms

Discussion

Patients undergoing heroin detoxification with methadone may feel that their withdrawal is proceeding too rapidly, and they may experience mild withdrawal effects. However, since a narcotic addict will often feel compelled to relate to others by requesting more drugs, and since withdrawal is not life-threatening, it is best to proceed on schedule in spite of patient demands. This contrasts with the best procedure for barbiturate withdrawal. An alternate method of withdrawing a patient from a narcotic is to allow the patient to determine the pace of withdrawal, with knowledge that the patient can only have a finite amount of methadone over a finite period of time. Such a withdrawal technique puts more responsibility on the patient. Patients being withdrawn from narcotics often engender anger in the physician, and punitive measures may be utilized, such as discharge, accusations of faking, and the use of a narcotic antagonist to "challenge the addiction." Obviously, none of these methods is appropriate.

7. If the patient remains in the hospital for complete detoxification, her chances of staying off of narcotics upon discharge are:
   A. Very good
   B. Good
   C. Fair
   D. Poor
8. Twenty years henceforth, it is likely that the patient will be:
   A. Using heroin
   B. Dead
   C. Not using heroin
   D. Suffering from a psychotic depression

Discussion

The short-term prognosis for remaining abstinent from heroin is very poor. Most patients return to using heroin within weeks to months after detoxification. However, the natural course of heroin addiction leads to cessation of heroin use as the patient ages. The long-term prognosis in this disorder is not particularly bad.

Answers

1. (C)
2. (B, C, D, E, and F)
5. (B)
6. (B and E)

3. (C)
4. (C)
7. (D)
8. (C)

References

1. Wesson, D. R. and Smith, D. E.: A conceptual approach to detoxification. *Journal of Psychedelic Drugs*, 6(2): 161–168, 1974.
2. Gruber, C. M., Jr., Stephens, V. C., and Terril, P. M.: Propoxyphene napsylate: Chemistry and experimental design. *Toxicology and Applied Pharmacology*, 19: 423–426, 1971.
3. Goldstein, A.: Heroin addiction and the role of methadone in its treatment. *Archives of General Psychiatry*, 26: 271–297, 1972.
4. Charney, D. S., Sternberg, D. E., Kleber, H. D., Heninger, G. R., and Redmond, E., Jr.: The clinical use of clonidine in abrupt withdrawal from methadone. *Archives of General Psychiatry*, 38: 1273–1277, 1981.

CASE 53: METHADONE MAINTENANCE THERAPY

A 32-year-old white laborer is admitted to a surgical unit for treatment of chronic osteomyelitis, which developed following an injury. The patient states that he has been involved in a methadone maintenance program for the past 10 months, explaining that it has been 16 hours since his last dose of methadone. He claims he has been given 50 mg per day of methadone in a single dose each morning. At the time you examine the patient, he demonstrates no evidence of discomfort. His pupils are equal in reaction to light and accommodation. There is no evidence of sweating, pilomotor erection, or rhinorrhea.

1. Methadone is used in the treatment of narcotic addicts, primarily because of its:
   A. Cross-tolerance with other opiate drugs
   B. Antagonism of opiate drugs
   C. Euphorogenic effect
   D. Sedative effect
   E. None of the above

Discussion

Chronically administered oral methadone, given in relatively high doses, does not appear to have a euphorogenic effect, but does induce a marked, slowly developing tolerance to all opiate-like drugs including methadone itself. As a result, a patient receiving methadone usually cannot experience the euphorogenic effects of ordinary doses of other narcotics, such as heroin and morphine. This then diminishes the rewarding or reinforcing effects of heroin or other abused narcotics.

2. The duration of action of methadone is usually:
   A. 4 hours
   B. 8 hours
   C. 12 hours
   D. 24 hours
   E. 48 hours
3. Signs of withdrawal from both heroin and methadone include all of the following except:
   A. Sweating
   B. Pilomotor erection
   C. Increase in pupil size
   D. Rhinorrhea
   E. Grand mal seizures

Discussion

Given daily, methadone, by virtue of its long duration of action (at least 24 hours), usually stabilizes the narcotic addict and prevents withdrawal. When methadone is withdrawn, signs of withdrawal are the same as those which occur with withdrawal from heroin and other narcotics, and include anxiety, pupillary dilation, rhinorrhea, sweating, and abdominal cramps. The probability that seizures will occur during narcotic withdrawal is very low. Should seizures occur during narcotic withdrawal, the possibility of concurrent addiction to alcohol or sedative–hypnotics should be considered, as should the possibility of a coexisting seizure disorder.

4. Compared to heroin withdrawal, the intensity of symptoms during methadone withdrawal is:
   A. Much less
   B. The same
   C. More severe
   D. Unrelated
5. One milligram of methadone is equivalent to:
   A. 3 mg morphine
   B. 1 mg heroin
   C. 20 mg meperidine (Demerol)
   D. 30 mg codeine
   E. All of the above

Discussion

The symptoms that occur with methadone withdrawal are more severe than those that occur with heroin withdrawal. Thus, when a patient is being withdrawn from methadone, such withdrawal should occur relatively slowly.

6. If surgery were required for this methadone maintenance patient, the preoperative management would require:
   A. Doubling the dose of methadone
   B. Continuing the current maintenance dose of methadone, with the last dose administered shortly before the anesthetic is given
   C. Switching to morphine during the patient's hospitalization
   D. Methadone is unnecessary, due to the suppressive effect of anesthesia
   E. Decreasing the methadone maintenance dose by 50%

Discussion

In the past decade, the number of addicts maintained on methadone who require surgery and anesthesia has increased. Severe withdrawal symptoms may be precipitated if the maintenance dosage of methadone is discontinued or replaced with inadequate preoperative narcotic medication. To prevent withdrawal reactions, the patient should receive the maintenance methadone dose prior to receiving an anesthetic.

Case Continued: Following surgery, the patient is transferred to another surgical unit. Thirty-six hours after surgery, you are called to consult because the patient has become very demanding of pain medications and is abusive, anxious, and angry. He has pilomotor erection, perspiration, rhinorrhea, and hyperactive bowel sounds.

7. With this clinical picture, it is likely that the patient is feigning withdrawal:
   A. True
   B. False

Case Continued: Review of the patient's chart reveals that no order for methadone now appears on it. You reinstitute methadone and the patient improves. Three days later the patient requests withdrawal from methadone, since he plans to travel to another country and will not be near a methadone program. He reiterates that he has been receiving methadone 50 mg per day.

8. To withdraw a patient from a 50 mg per day methadone habit, the first written order should be:
   A. 30 mg methadone per day
   B. 20 mg methadone every 8 hours
   C. 10 mg methadone every 12 hours
   D. 20 mg methadone every 12 hours
9. Most patients can be detoxified by decreasing the total daily dose by the following amount during each 24-hour period:
   A. 5 mg
   B. 10 mg
   C. 15 mg
   D. 5 mg every other day
10. On the second day of detoxification, the patient appears to have mild anorexia, anxiety, and muscle aches. This suggests that you have been decreasing the methadone too rapidly:
   A. True
   B. False

Discussion

Narcotics addicts often feel they are not receiving enough drug during detoxification. However, it is best to set a withdrawal sequence lasting 6 to 10 days and rigidly adhere to this program. Minor tranquilizers, tricyclic antidepressants, and anticholinergics may be helpful in making the patient more comfortable.

11. The best way to determine the specific dose of methadone necessary to stabilize a given patient prior to detoxification is to:
    A. Ask the patient how much heroin he uses
    B. Ask the patient how much discomfort he is feeling
    C. Hold all medications until there are severe signs of withdrawal such as diarrhea, vomiting, or cramps
    D. Observe for mild objective signs of withdrawal, such as pilomotor erection, and give enough methadone to suppress these
12. The best route for administering methadone is:
    A. Tablet
    B. Syrup
    C. Injection
13. To determine a daily beginning methadone dose prior to detoxification, the initial methadone dose should be:
    A. 5 mg methadone
    B. 10 mg methadone
    C. 15 mg methadone
    D. 20 mg methadone
14. This initial methadone dose should be repeated at 4- to 6-hour intervals:
    A. As a matter of routine
    B. If objective clinical signs of gastrointestinal hyperactivity, mydriasis, rhinorrhea, or pilomotor erection continue
    C. Until the patient is somnolent
15. Which of the following substances, taken in high doses, can produce seizures?
    A. Heroin
    B. Codeine
    C. Methadone
    D. Meperidine (Demerol)

Discussion

Complaints, hostility, irritability, immaturity, grumbling, and feigning illness are very common during opiate withdrawal. Even perspiring and rhinorrhea can be faked by skilled individuals. More objective signs of withdrawal, such as pilomotor erection and mydriasis, are more reliable in assessing whether or not an individual is in narcotics withdrawal. Since opiate addicts often exaggerate the amount of drug they have been taking, an accurate estimate by interview is often impossible. The initial dosage of methadone needed to stabilize an addict prior to withdrawal should be based on the amount of methadone needed to prevent moderate to severe signs of abstinence, such as vomiting, diarrhea, febrile states, and severe cramping; and physiologic signs of withdrawal, such as goose flesh and mydriasis. It is rare for any addict to require more than 40 mg methadone during a 24-hour period. Deaths due to overdosing by excessive methadone have been reported in hospitalized addicts. They may occur because a patient fakes symptoms and obtains too much methadone. The addict should be told to expect some discomfort during the detoxification. It may be helpful to suggest that the more that symptoms are experienced, the more rapidly the syndrome will end and detoxification will be completed. A firm, supportive, but uncompromising attitude is most effective in allaying anxiety and dealing with the regressed immaturity and demanding hostility characteristic of the narcotic-withdrawal syndrome. Once the symptoms of withdrawal are controlled (this usually requires approximately 30 to 40 mg methadone every 24 hours), the methadone dosage may be decreased by 10 mg every 24 hours (5 mg every 12 hours). Should a debilitating medical or surgical illness coexist, the dosage should be decreased by 5 mg per 24 hours to minimize difficulties. When a patient is being stabilized on methadone prior to detoxification, or is being detoxified, methadone is best given in syrup form. This prevents "cheeking" a tablet or giving the patient the reinforcement of receiving an injection. Symptoms occurring during detoxification that are uncharacteristic of opiate withdrawal must alert the physician to the possibility that the patient is addicted to other drugs (i.e., barbiturates, other sedative hypnotics, alcohol) or that the patient has medical complications such as endocarditis or hepatitis. The only opiate-related drug which, in large doses, can produce seizures is meperidine.

Answers

1. (A)
2. (D)
3. (E)
4. (C)
5. (E)
6. (B)
7. (B)
8. (D)
9. (B)
10. (B)
11. (D)
12. (B)
13. (B)
14. (B)
15. (D)

References

1. Goldstein, A.: Heroin addiction and the role of methadone in its treatment. *Archives of General Psychiatry*, 26: 271–297, 1972.
2. Blackly, P. H.: Management of the opiate abstinence syndrome. *American Journal of Psychiatry*, 122:742, 1966.
3. DiMascio, A. and Shader, R. I. (eds.): *Clinical Handbook of Psychopharmacology*. Jason Aronson, New York, 1970, p. 251.

CASE 54: TREATMENT OF PAIN IN A TERMINALLY ILL PATIENT

You are asked to see a 48-year-old white male accountant who has been admitted with end-stage metastatic adenocarcinoma of the large bowel. His internist has followed the patient for 2 years, and has most recently been concerned because of significant problems with pain. There has been no history of mental illness. Over the past 6 months the patient has had an increasing need for pain medications. There have been metastatic lesions noted in the region of the lung, and there is a suspicion of some bone metastasis, although definitive radiographic evidence has been unsupportive and bone scans are somewhat inconclusive.

1. The patient with chronic pain should have clear-cut objective evidence, represented by hyperactive autonomic nervous system dysfunction, to characterize the pain syndrome:

A. True
B. False

2. The most important category to consider relative to pain in a patient with cancer is:
   A. Pain syndromes associated with direct tumor infiltration or metastasis
   B. Pain syndromes associated with cancer therapy
   C. Pain syndromes unassociated with cancer or cancer therapy

Discussion

Acute and chronic pain states present differently. Acute pain is the easier to recognize because of a hyperactive autonomic (i.e., sympathetic) nervous system. Patients with chronic pain that has persisted for days to weeks, although they may complain of and experience agonizing discomfort, may have very little objective evidence of such a state (e.g., sympathetic signs). Hyperactive autonomic nervous system dysfunction is not usually present, and this might mislead the examiner to believe that a psychogenic factor is at work. The most important category of cancer pain is associated with direct tumor infiltration or metastasis, and is responsible for the majority of pain-associated problems in both the inpatient and outpatient cancer patient population. Pain associated with cancer therapy itself is approximately one-third to one-fourth as common, and pain associated with unrelated causes, such as disc disease and arthritis, may occur in only 3 to 10% of cases.

3. Pain perception is simply a function of the amount of tissue damage sustained by the patient:
   A. True
   B. False

Discussion

Pain perception is not simply a function of the amount of tissue damage sustained by the patient, but reflects a variety of factors including age, sex, underlying personality, previous history of painful experiences, cultural expectations, and secondary gain as a result of caring and sympathy received and time off from work.

4. The most effective intervention in the dying patient with severe pain should be:
   A. Working through earlier psychological factors in regard to conflict
   B. Careful limitation of pain medications to prevent addiction
   C. Control of pain as necessary to prevent suffering

Discussion

Maintenance of the integrity of personality in the face of demoralizing pain presents a severe challenge to the physician. Inadequate control of pain in dying patients exacerbates the suffering and damages a care-giving relationship, as well as the relationship between the family and the patient. The risk–benefit ratio of an analgesic strategy, such as the risk of addiction, should be less important than pain reduction in the dying patient. An especially complicated problem occurs in the case of patients who have been very demanding and complaining and who are thus especially vulnerable to inadequate pain medication.

5. In the patient described above, medication should be provided on an as-needed basis:
   A. True
   B. False

Discussion

Medication for severe cancer pain in dying patients should be administered on a standardized and predetermined around-the-clock basis. Analgesics that have been ordered on an as-needed basis frequently do not provide optimal pain relief. Difficulty with the prompt administration of medication by a busy staff, as well as reluctance on the part of some patients to ask for medication, complicates effective and smooth pain management in cancer.

6. Match the following medications with their effective durations:

A. Morphine 1. 120 minutes

B. Oxycodone 2. 180 minutes
C. Methadone 3. 240 minutes
D. Codeine 4. 360 minutes

7. In patients receiving pain-killing drugs with a relatively longer plasma half-life, such as methadone and levorphanol:
   A. There is no difficulty with cross-tolerance
   B. Patients can receive these medications relatively infrequently
   C. Repeated administration of these drugs can lead to excessive sedation and respiratory depression.
   D. B and C

Discussion

Intervals between doses of a pain-killing drug depend upon the individual's particular physiological capacity for utilization and excretion of the drug. Opiate-naive patients or inpatients with hepatic–renal dysfunction can easily have excessive sedation and respiratory depression, especially when drugs with long plasma half-lives are used. Incomplete cross-tolerance between drugs also necessitates caution when one changes from a drug to which the patient has become tolerant to a new agent.

8. Which of the following symptoms characterize the syndrome seen upon the abrupt withdrawal of medication in patients who have been chronically treated with narcotic analgesics?
   A. Tremor
   B. Insomnia
   C. Autonomic nervous system excitability
   D. Agitation
   E. All of the above

Discussion

Agitation, tremor, insomnia, and autonomic nervous system excitability are representative of the acute and abrupt withdrawal of narcotic medications. By slowly tapering the dose of medication, the appearance of abstinence symptoms is less likely. Reinstituting the drug at 25% of the previous daily dose suppresses these symptoms.

9. Match the following categories and medications:
   A. Chlorpromazine
   B. Phenytoin
   C. Corticosteroids
   D. Amitriptyline
   (1) Anticonvulsant action stabilizes neuronal membranes by suppressing spontaneous firing, lessening pain especially in neuronally sensitive areas
   (2) Antiemetic and antianxiety properties
   (3) Analgesic mechanism of action related to ability to enhance serotonin activity in the central nervous system
   (4) Especially used for reducing pain from metastatic bone lesions, and has the capacity to enhance mood and appetite as well

Discussion

Anticonvulsants have proven useful in managing pain problems in which there is neuronal sensitivity, such as phantom limb pain and neuromas. The phenothiazines have been shown to have only a minimal analgesic effect, but are especially useful in alleviating significant anxiety and emetic problems. The sedative and mood-enhancing effects of antidepressants may be of great use in patients with severe cancer pain. Dexamethasone is commonly used in divided doses of 10 to 20 mg, especially in patients who have severe bone metastases, and may also be of assistance when there is poor appetite and dysphoria. Corticosteroids, however, have often been shown to be effective only for short-term use, owing to the rapid development of resistance to their analgesic effects and other complications with regard to glucose intolerance and secondary infection.

Answers

1. (B)
2. (A)
3. (B)
4. (C)
5. (B)
6. (A-2, B-3, C-4, D-3)
7. (D)
8. (E)
9. (A-2, B-1, C-4, D-3)

References

1. Moulin, D. E. and Foley, K.: Management of pain in patients with cancer. *Psychiatric Annals*, 14(11): 815–822, 1984.
2. Foley, K. N.: The management of pain of malignant origin. In: *Current Neurology*, Vol 2 (eds.: H. R. Tyler and D. M. Dawson). Houghton Mifflin, Boston, 1979, pp. 279–302.
3. Twycross, R. G.: Pain in far advanced cancer. *Pain*, 14: 303–310, 1982.
4. Walsh, T. C.: Antidepressants in chronic pain. *Clinical Neuropharmacology*, 6: 271–295, 1983.

CASE 55: TREATMENT OF AN ADVERSE LYSERGIC ACID DIETHYLAMIDE (LSD) REACTION

A 19-year-old white man presents in the emergency room as delusional, hallucinatory, agitated, and frightened, yet oriented and alert. He has dilated pupils and states that he took a "hit" of lysergic acid diethylamide (LSD) 1 hour prior to admission. His friends announce that this is true and that he is having a "bad trip."

1. The treatment of choice for this patient includes:
   A. An antipsychotic drug such as chlorpromazine (Thorazine)
   B. Diazepam (Valium)
   C. Reassurance
   D. Scopolamine
2. The panic reaction will most likely last:
   A. 12 to 24 hours
   B. 24 to 48 hours
   C. 48 to 72 hours
   D. 72 hours to 1 week
3. The psychotic symptoms may last for:
   A. No longer than the acute effect of the LSD
   B. Months or years
   C. A and B
   D. Neither A nor B

Discussion

An LSD panic reaction usually lasts from 12 to 24 hours and then disappears. However, in patients with pre-existing schizophrenic illness or severe borderline characteristics, LSD may precipitate a lasting psychosis. The treatment of choice for an LSD-induced panic state or "bad trip" is to offer reassurance and contact, and to give diazepam or another antianxiety drug. Although the phenothiazines are remarkably effective in counteracting LSDs central effects, they are not advised in treating LSD-induced "bad trips." This is true because what is thought to be LSD may actually be scopolamine or another hallucinogen such as phencyclidine (PCP), which reacts adversely with a phenothiazine or other antipsychotic agent. In general, the patient should not be left alone or unobserved, especially if PCP abuse is suspected, since these patients may hurt themselves or others, or attempt suicide.

Answers

1. (B and C)
2. (A)
3. (C)

References

1. Lisansky, J., Strassman, R., Janowsky, D. S., and Risch, S. C.: Drug induced psychoses. In: *Transient Psychoses* (eds.: J. Tupin, J. Pena, and U. Halbreich). Brunner/Mazel, New York, 1984, pp. 80–110.

CASE 56: SEDATIVE–HYPNOTIC DETOXIFICATION

A 23-year-old black female patient has a 3-year history of intermittent polydrug abuse. She has taken psychostimulants, hallucinogens, and sedative–hypnotics. She reports that for the past 4 months she has been taking 10 to 15 secobarbital (Seconal) tablets per day, and is taking amphetamines to wake up in the morning.

1. The patient's physical symptoms most likely include:
   A. Ataxia, lateral nystagmus, and dysarthria
   B. Hypotension, a pill-rolling tremor, and salivation
   C. Dilated pupils, diaphoresis, and increased blood pressure
2. The patient's emotional symptoms most likely include:
   A. Emotional lability
   B. Hyperalertness
   C. Anergy
   D. Constant euphoria
3. Medical management of the patient's symptoms involves:
   A. Discontinuing barbiturates immediately
   B. Tapering the barbiturate dosage over a 3-day period
   C. Intoxicating the patient on barbiturates and then tapering the dosage over a 12- to 14-day period, with adjustment of the schedule if withdrawal symptoms occur
   D. Consistently decreasing the patient's barbiturates over a 14-day period and not changing the drug schedule regardless of the appearance of withdrawal symptoms
4. Barbiturate withdrawal should be performed in:
   A. An outpatient setting
   B. An Inpatient setting
   C. Self-help group

Discussion

It is quite likely that the patient is addicted to barbiturates. A patient can become addicted to approximately 600 mg per day of secobarbital or its equivalent. Similarly, methaqualone (Quaalude) can addict a person at doses within the therapeutic range. This patient is typical of young "street-culture" drug abusers in that she has used multiple drugs at different times for nonmedical purposes. Barbiturate and sedative–hypnotic addicts usually present with a symptom complex consisting of emotional lability, irritability, lateral nystagmus, ataxia, dysarthria, and elevated serum barbiturate or sedative hypnotic levels. Abrupt withdrawal of sedative hypnotics in addicted individuals can lead to severe withdrawal symptoms, which are similar to delirium tremens. Patients initially show insomnia, anxiety, tachycardia, and hyptertension. Later they may develop an organic brain syndrome with confusion, visual and auditory hallucinations, agitation, seizures, and hyperpyrexia. Appropriate treatment of barbiturate or sedative-hypnotic addiction consists of slowly tapering a patient's dosage over a period of about 2 weeks. If withdrawal symptoms occur or recur during the withdrawal period, the barbiturate dose should be increased to an intoxicating level and withdrawal should then proceed. It is best to perform barbiturate withdrawal in an inpatient setting, since this withdrawal is a medically serious problem, and since it is difficult for barbiturate addicts to exercise self control in abstaining from barbiturates while withdrawing from them.

Answers

1. (A)
2. (A)
3. (C)
4. (B)

References

1. Wesson, D. R. and Smith, D. E.: A conceptual approach to detoxification. *Journal of Psychedelic Drugs*, 6: 161–168, 1974.
2. Smith, D. E. and Wesson, D. R.: Phenobarbital technique in treatment of barbiturate dependence. *Archives of General Psychiatry*, 24: 56–60, 1971.
3. Freedman, A. M. and Kaplan, A. E.: *Comprehensive Textbook of Psychiatry*, Vol. 2. Williams and Wilkins, Baltimore, 1976, pp. 1327–1329.
4. Wikler, A.: Diagnosis and treatment of drug dependence of barbiturate type. *American Journal of Psychiatry*, 125: 758, 1968.

SECTION VI
DISORDERS OF CHILDHOOD

CASE 57: TREATMENT OF ENURESIS

The patient is an 11-year-old boy brought to your office for evaluation of bedwetting during sleep. The mother relates that the bedwetting has been a lifelong difficulty for the boy. The bedwetting occurs, on the average, every other night. Enuresis has caused the patient a great deal of emotional stress, as he is currently in a Scout troop and this problem prevents him from participating in field trips and camping activities due to his fears of embarrassment. A routine urinalysis and blood count are both within normal limits.

1. Operationally, enuresis can be defined as bedwetting or clothes-wetting in persons over the age of:
   A. 24 months
   B. 3 years
   C. 5 years
   D. 7 years
   E. 12 years

Discussion

Individuals over the age of 3, who fail to inhibit the urge to urinate during the waking hours or during sleep, can be considered enuretic. During the school years, 16% of children are enuretic after age 5; by age 7½, only 7% are enuretic. Between 7½ years and 18 years, the percentage of enuretics in the general population drops to about 2%.

2. Factors suggesting an associated or causative organic pathology in enuretic patients include:
   A. Presence of urinary frequency and urgency
   B. Nocturnal enuresis exclusively
   C. Daytime enuresis

Discussion

The prevalence of an organic etiology in patients with enuresis varies from 1% to 10%. Patients who are enuretic only at night are much less likely to have any associated organic pathology. Eighty percent of enuretics have episodes only at night. Fifteen percent have daytime and nocturnal episodes. Five percent are daytime enuretics only. The physician must be especially aware of the possibility of an organic etiology in this last group. Symptoms consistent with bladder and kidney disease, such as frequency and urgency, necessitate a complete pediatric and urological examination.

3. For those patients who have enuresis extending into adolescence, there is a greater frequency of all the following except for:
   A. Past history of sleepwalking
   B. Inferior dentition
   C. Chronic genitourinary-tract complaints
   D. Psychological disturbances predisposing to enuresis
   E. Family history of enuresis
4. The following factors are important in the pathophysiology of enuresis:
   A. Genitourinary-tract factors
   B. Sleep-physiology factors
   C. Water-regulation factors
   D. All of the above
   E. None of the above

Discussion

Besides overt genitourinary-tract disease, covert pathology, such as a small functional bladder capacity or a deficit in neurological control of micturition and a developmental lag may be factors which cause enuresis. It has long been noted that bedwetters are heavy sleepers and studies have revealed that bladder filling during sleep is most crucial in enuresis. Compared to controls, the enuretic has an increased frequency of bladder contractions, which are prominent just prior to micturition.

5. Enuresis as the result of psychological conflict is felt to occur in:
   A. 80% of cases
   B. 60% of cases
   C. 40% of cases
   D. 20% of cases
   E. 5% of cases

Discussion

A neurotic conflict such as the birth of a sibling, or a transient emotional stress such as making the adjustment to military service, may precipitate enuresis. In these cases, enuresis is a regressive phenomenon and psychological factors should be explored as its cause.

6. The drug of choice in the treatment of enuresis is:
   A. Tincture of belladonna
   B. Phenobarbital
   C. Diphenhydramine hydrochloride
   D. Imipramine
   E. Chlorpromazine

Discussion

Over 100 investigations have shown that imipramine is superior to placebo in decreasing the frequency of bedwetting. The usual daily dosage for a 6- to 12-year-old child is 25 mg, although some children may require as much as 75 mg. However, the institution of imipramine as a treatment for enuresis should be weighed carefully, owing to the side effects of this drug.

7. The effective imipramine dosing schedule for enuresis is:
   A. Three times daily
   B. At bedtime
   C. 8 hours before bedtime
   D. Upon morning awakening
   E. None of the above

Discussion

There is evidence that if a child wets his bed prior to 1:00 A.M., he should receive his medication around 3:00 P.M. If, however, enuresis usually occurs after 1:00 A.M., the medication should be given at about 8:00 P.M. For many adults and children, antidepressant medications given at bedtime produce good results, and this is by far the most commonly used dosage schedule. However, there should be flexibility in each individual case.

8. The enuretic patient should be kept on imipramine for the following period, after which the medication should be withdrawn over a 4-week period:
   A. 2 weeks
   B. 8 weeks
   C. 12 weeks
   D. 1 year
   E. 2 years

Discussion

It has been suggested that after a 6- to 8-week trial of imipramine, withdrawal should occur over a period of 4 weeks. If bedwetting returns, imipramine or other tricyclic antidepressants should once again be tried.

9. Overall, the percent of expected improvement of enuresis with imipramine treatment is:
   A. 10% fewer wet nights
   B. 30% fewer wet nights

C. 60% fewer wet nights
D. 80% fewer wet nights
E. 95% fewer wet nights

Discussion

A double-blind study of 57 children (aged 5 to 15) with nocturnal enuresis occurring at least 3 nights per week for more than 6 months demonstrated that dosages between 10 and 25 mg imipramine pamoate at bedtime reduced the frequency of enuresis by 60%.

10. The most likely mechanism of action of imipramine's effectiveness in enuresis is:
    A. Anticholinergic effects on bladder capacity
    B. The antidepressant effect of the drug
    C. Central-nervous-system effects on sleep patterns
    D. Direct anesthetic effect on bladder musculature

Discussion

Most investigators have implicated imipramine's central-nervous-system-stimulating effects on sleep patterns as the principal causes of its efficacy in enuresis. Imipramine's parasympatholytic and atropine-like effect may relax the detrusor muscle of the urinary bladder, decrease the irritability of the bladder musculature, and abolish the involuntary contractions of the immature bladder. However, noncentrally acting anticholinergic agents are not antineuretic agents.

Answers

1. (B)
2. (A and C)
3. (D)
4. (D)
5. (D)
6. (D)
7. (E)
8. (B)
9. (C)
10. (C)

References

1. Klackenberg, G.: A prospective longitudinal study of children: Data on psychic health and development up to eight years of age. *Acta Pediatrica Scandinavica* (Supplement) 224: 210–225, 1971.
2. Martin, C. R. A.: *A New Approach to Nocturnal Enuresis*. Lewis, London, 1966.
3. Arena, J. M. (ed.): *Complete Pediatrician*, Vol. 9. Lea and Febiger, Philadelphia, 1969.
4. Baker, B.: Symptom treatment and symptom substitution in enuresis. *Journal of Abnormal Psychology*, 74: 42, 1969.
5. Broughton, R. J.: Sleep disorders, enuresis, somnambulism, and nightmares occur in confusional states of arousal, not in "dreaming sleep." *Science*, 159: 1070, 1968.
6. MacLean, R. E. G.: Imipramine hydrochloride (Tofranil) and enuresis. *American Journal of Psychiatry*, 117: 551, 1960.
7. Gilbert, I. and Martin, G. I.: Imipramine pamoate in the treatment of childhood enuresis, a double-blind study. *American Journal of Diseases of Children*, 122: 42–47, 1971.
8. Zung, W. K.: Effect of antidepressant drugs on sleeping and dreaming. *Excerpta Medica International Foundation Congress, Series*, 150: 1824–1825, 1968.
9. Ditman, K. S. and Blinn, K. A.: Sleep levels in enuresis. *American Journal of Psychiatry*, 111: 115–120, 1965.
10. Rapoport, J. L., Mikkelsen, E. J., Zavadil, A., *et al.*: Childhood enuresis: II. Psychopathology, tricyclic concentration in plasma, and antienuretic effect. *Archives of General Psychiatry*, 37: 1146–1152, 1980.
11. Law, W., Petti, T. A., and Kazdin, A. E.: Withdrawal symptoms after graduated cessation of imipramine in children. *American Journal of Psychiatry*, 138(5): 647–650, 1981.
12. Blau, S.: A guide to the use of psychotropic medications in children and adolescents. *Journal of Clinical Psychiatry*, 39: 766–772, 1978.

CASE 58: TREATMENT OF GILLES DE LA TOURETTE SYNDROME

An 8-year-old white boy, brought in by his parents, has shown progressive deterioration in behavior over the preceding year. The parents state that the boy has shown periodic grimacing and quick movements of the upper part of his body. His activity comes in bursts, during which time he will hop, skip, or jump. This often occurs at inappropriate times such as at family gatherings. Over the past few months the patient's symptoms have included swearing and the utterance of obscenities, indiscriminately shouted with obvious conversational intent. The strange behavior is exhibited spontaneously and unpredictably, and has been found to worsen with the recent stress of returning to school. Examination of the patient reveals signs and symptoms consistent with the history given by the patient's parents. Tic-like actions, including hopping, skipping, grinding of teeth, and sudden compulsive motor outbursts are apparent. The patient attempts to relate in a social manner. However, at times he seems compelled to swear and to utter obscenities. There do not appear to be hallucinations or delusions.

1. The most probable diagnosis for this patient is:
   A. Huntington's chorea
   B. Childhood schizophrenia
   C. Hyperactive syndrome of childhood
   D. Gilles de la Tourette syndrome
   E. Wilson's disease
2. With stress, the symptoms of this syndrome usually show:
   A. Improvement
   B. Worsening
   C. No change
   D. All of the above
3. The utterance of obscenities or involuntary guttural sounds is called:
   A. Cataplexy
   B. Catalepsy
   C. Coprolalia
   D. Enuresis
   E. Encopresis
4. The illness most likely has an organic basis:
   A. True
   B. False
5. The illness has been shown to definitely have the following features, in addition to motor disturbance:
   A. Obsessive–compulsive traits

B. Heightened hostility
C. Hypochondriasis
D. A tendency toward psychosis
E. All of the above
F. None of the above

6. "Soft" neurological signs, such as nonspecific electroencephalographic (EEG) findings, indicating central nervous system abnormalities, are observed in:
A. 10% of these patients
B. 25% of these patients
C. 50% of these patients
D. 80% of these patients
E. 95% of these patients

Discussion

In 1885 Gilles de la Tourette first described an illness appearing in children between the ages of 2 and 12 years. Patients with this illness demonstrate a repertoire of motor tics that involves spasmodic movements of the upper part of the body, spreading to the rest of the body, with compulsive coprolalia accompanying these muscular tics. These coprolalic verbalizations are present in approximately 50% of cases. The strange behavior exhibited is usually spontaneous and unpredictable, although it may be triggered or made worse when the patient is experiencing emotional stress or fatigue. In making the diagnosis of Gilles de la Tourette syndrome, degenerative diseases of the central nervous system must be ruled out. One-half of patients with Gilles de la Tourette syndrome demonstrate EEG and neurological abnormalities, but these are usually benign.

7. Current evidence suggests that the principal causative factor of Gilles de la Tourette syndrome is hyperactivity of the:
A. Adrenergic system
B. Dopaminergic system
C. Cholinergic system
D. Serotonergic system
E. None of the above

Discussion

Theories about the etiology of Gilles de la Tourette syndrome have ranged from a proposed functional origin to a specific organic deficit. Shapiro *et al.* evaluated 34 patients with this syndrome on a psychiatric and psychological basis. They found that obsessive–compulsive traits were infrequent, inhibition of hostilities was not prominent, hysteria and hypochondriasis were not characteristic, and schizophrenia was not present. Intelligence quotients of patients with this disease are not different from those of the general population, and their personality structure does not seem to be impaired. Shapiro *et al.* concluded that the cause of Gilles de la Tourette syndrome is a disorder of the central nervous system. Others have proposed that hyperactivity of the dopaminergic system is the principal causative factor.

8. To date, the most effective drug for treating the syndrome has been:
   A. Diazepam (Valium)
   B. Chlorpromazine (Thorazine)
   C. Imipramine (Tofranil)
   D. Haloperidol (Haldol)
   E. Phenobarbital

Discussion

Haloperidol (Haldol) is the drug of choice in the treatment of Gilles de la Tourette syndrome. Prior studies show few favorable results with insulin treatment, sedatives, muscle relaxants, conditioning therapy, and hypnosis. Some modest success was found with long-term supportive psychotherapy for the patient and his family. Doses of haloperidol of 6 to 180 mg per day may be required to control symptoms of the syndrome, and most patients show more than a 90% reduction in their symptoms after 1 year of treatment. Haloperidol is a difficult drug to use, in that its many side effects and the spontaneous waxing and waning of symptoms in Gilles de la Tourette syndrome demand careful monitoring and continued careful adjustment of the dose. Medication should be started at a low dose, and improvement as well as the development of side effects noted. The peculiar response of this syndrome to megadoses of haloperidol suggests a careful but thorough clinical trial of haloperidol before treatment is abandoned.

Answers

1. (D)	5. (F)
2. (B)	6. (C)
3. (C)	7. (B)
4. (A)	8. (D)

References

1. Brunn, R. D. and Shapiro, A. K.: Differential diagnosis of the Gilles de la Tourette Syndrome. *Journal of Nervous and Mental Disorders*, 155: 328, 1972.
2. Morpew, J. A. and Sim, M.: Gilles de la Tourette syndrome: A clinical and psychopathological study. *British Journal of Medical Psychology*, 42: 293, 1969.
3. Shapiro, A. K., Shapiro, E., and Wayne, H.: Birth, developmental, and family history in demographic information in Tourette syndrome. *Journal of Nervous and Mental Disease*, 155: 335, 1973.
4. Friel, P. B.: Familial incidence of Gilles de la Tourette syndrome, with observation on etiology and treatment. *British Journal of Psychiatry*, 122: 655, 1975.
5. Eisenberg, L., Ascher, E., and Kanner, L.: A clinical study of Gilles de la Tourette syndrome in children. *American Journal of Psychiatry*, 155: 715, 1959.
6. Shapiro, A. K., Shapiro, E., and Wayne, H.: Treatment of Tourette's syndrome. *Archives of General Psychiatry*, 28: 92, 1973.
7. Borison, R. L., Ang, L., Chang, S., *et al.*: New pharmacological approaches in the treatment of Tourette syndrome (Gilles de la Tourette syndrome). *Advances in Neurology*, 35: 377–382, 1982.
8. Campel, M., Cohen, I., and Anderson, L.: Pharmacotherapy for autistic children: A summary of research. *American Journal of Psychiatry*, 26: 265–273, June 1981.
9. Gualtieri, C. T., Barnhill, J., McGimsey, J., *et al.*: Tardive dyskinesia and other movement disorders in children treated with psychotropic drugs. *Journal of the American Academy of Child Psychiatry*, 19(3): 491–510, 1980.

10. Blau, S.: A guide to the use of psychotropic medication in children and adolescents. *Journal of Clinical Psychiatry*, 39: 766–772, 1978.
11. Aman, M.: Drugs, learning and the phenothiazines. In: *Pediatric Psychopharmacology: The Use of Behavior Modifying Drugs in Children* (ed.: J. S. Werry). Brunner/Mazel, New York, 1978.

CASE 59: TREATMENT OF HYPERKINETIC CHILD SYNDROME

The patient is a 9-year-old boy who is brought to your office for evaluation. The mother is extremely concerned by his progressive inability to function appropriately in the classroom. His teachers have told her that the patient is unable to control his level of motor activity. He is said to have trouble concentrating and is "fidgety." The patient's mother states that he has always been a restless child, and that while her other children were able to routinely nap or focus on single activities, the patient was easily distracted, unable to complete tasks, and always calling for attention. The mother further states that the patient has always been a difficult child to manage, taking infrequent and short naps, having continued discipline problems, running into the street in spite of continued warnings, and climbing trees in the neighborhood in spite of her admonitions. When disciplined, he has become extremely angry and gone into temper tantrums. He has fights with his siblings over trivial matters. The patient's mother states that his school performance has been below average. However, with considerable tutoring on her part he has maintained an adequate position in his class, although below the level attained by his three older siblings.

1. The diagnosis that best describes this patient's difficulties is probably:
   A. Schizophrenia, childhood type
   B. Overanxious reaction of childhood
   C. Transient adjustment reaction of childhood
   D. Mental retardation
   E. Attention deficit disorder of childhood

Discussion

Attention deficit disorder (ADD), associated with or without minimal brain dysfunction (MBD), is probably the single most common disorder seen by child psychiatrists. Hyperactivity is a nonspecific symptom complex, and not a personality disorder as such. It is considered a sign of developmental immaturity only when it persists after the age of 7, or when it occurs to an excessive degree. Manifestations of the hyperkinetic state change with age. Some children, almost from birth, have colic and are restless. Parental prohibitions are usually without significant effect. Terms such as "brain damage syndrome," "minimal brain damage," and "minimal brain dysfunction" are often used synonomously with the term "hyperactive child syndrome." These terms are somewhat misleading in that frank brain damage is not present in the majority of hyperactive children, and alternately, most brain-damaged children do not present with the hyperactive child syndrome. Depression must be considered in the differential diagnosis of the hyperactive state.

2. Besides hyperactivity, other cardinal features of the clinical picture in attention deficit disorder include:
   A. Distractability
   B. Impulsivity
   C. Excitability
   D. Antisocial behavior

Discussion

Distractability is most noticeable in the school situation, but is usually also reported by parents. It is when the hyperactive child reaches the school system that the diagnosis is most often and most easily made. Behaviors that are disturbing but tolerated in the home situation are not so easily tolerated in the classroom setting. Impulsivity is shown by such behaviors as jumping into the deep end of the swimming pool without knowing how to swim, running into the street in front of cars, climbing onto high roof tops and ledges, and blurting out tactless statements. Excitability is manifested by temper tantrums and fights over trivial matters, a low frustration tolerance, and a tendency to become over-excited and more active in stimulating situations, such as in large groups of children. Therefore, hyperactivity, distractability, impulsivity, and excitability are considered the cardinal symptoms of the hyperkinetic syndrome. Other symptoms are often seen, but are not necessarily associated with the syndrome. Aggressive and antisocial behavior, cognitive and learning disabilities, and emotional symptoms such as depression and low self-esteem may point toward additional or associated disorders, but are not primary to the hyperkinetic syndrome.

3. Before a definitive diagnosis of hyperactivity syndrome can be made, the following diagnostic signs must be evident:
   A. A low IQ on testing
   B. Evidence of frank brain damage through the demonstration of "soft neurological signs"
   C. A family history of psychiatrically disturbed parents
   D. Electroencephalographic abnormalities
   E. None of these

Discussion

Although any one of the above symptoms may be associated with the diagnosis of attention deficit disorder, the diagnosis describes a heterogenous group of children. In some cases the disorder may be due to a structural abnormality of the brain. In others there may be an abnormality of physiological arousal of the nervous system. In many children no abnormalities are evident. In addition, clinical studies of the parents of children with the hyperactivity syndrome indicate that a significant percentage were themselves hyperactive as children and are psychiatrically disturbed as adults. Another study indicates that adults who were previously hyperkinetic respond positively to psychostimulants, such as methylphenidate.

4. The class of pharmacologic agents most effective in the hyperkinetic syndrome is:
   A. The stimulants
   B. The antidepressants
   C. The antianxiety agents
   D. The antihistamines
   E. The phenothiazines

Discussion

The stimulants methylphenidate (Ritalin), pemoline (Cylert), and dextroamphetamine (Desoxyn) have been shown to be effective in two-thirds to three-fourths of behaviorally defined hyperkinetic children. These stimulants produce a decrease in hyperactivity and impulsivity and an increase in attention span. The rather large literature on the use of major and minor tranquilizers in hyperkinetic states consists largely of uncontrolled studies and contradictory findings, although there is general agreement that the major tranquilizers produce deleterious effects on learning and cognitive functioning. Although the antihistamine known as diphenhydramine has been advocated in treating hyperkinetic children, it has not been proven useful in controlled comparative studies. However, it may represent a useful drug for alternative attempts at control. Tricyclic antidepressants have been found effective by some investigators and not nearly as effective as methylphenidate by other investigators. In addition, lithium carbonate and the anticonvulsants have been used to treat hyperkinetic children, with varying success. There is no evidence that anticonvulsants are indicated for hyperactive children with abnormal EEGs and in the absence of seizures.

5. You have decided to begin the patient on stimulant medications and to follow him on a weekly basis at your office. Your choice(s) initially would be:
   A. Dextroamphetamine 15 mg, b.i.d.
   B. Dextroamphetamine 5 mg, b.i.d.
   C. Dextroamphetamine 10 mg, at bedtime
   D. Methylphenidate 10 mg, b.i.d.
   E. Methylphenidate 30 mg, in the morning
   F. Pemoline 37.5 mg every morning

Discussion

Dosages of 0.5 mg/kg methylphenidate, or 0.25 mg/kg dextroamphetamine, or 37.5 mg pemoline often are effective in treating the hyperkinetic syndrome. The dosage schedule should be such that the drugs are taken during the periods of greatest activity, such as during mornings and afternoons. Evening dosing would therefore usually be less effective.

6. The effectiveness of stimulants will be seen in:
   A. 2 to 6 hours
   B. 1 week
   C. 3 weeks
   D. 8 weeks

Discussion

The latency of onset of action for both methylphenidate and dextroamphetamine is approximately 30 minutes, with a 3- to 6-hour duration of action. Methylphenidate must be given at least twice a day to insure effectiveness throughout the school day. If dextroamphetamine is given in long-acting spansule form, it need be only given once a day. Pemoline is given once per day in the morning. Its dosage may need to be increased to 56.25 to 75 mg per day. Response to treatment is probably singly best evaluated from behavioral changes at school. It is said that if the stimulant is effective at all, rapid results will be seen.

Case Continued: You put the patient on dextroamphetamine 5.0 mg, b.i.d. The patient's mother calls you after 3 days and states that although there has been some minimal improvement, she feels that the patient has not responded to the drug as she had hoped.

7. Your next decision should be to:
   A. Stop the stimulants and observe the patient
   B. Stop the stimulants and put the patient on diphenhydramine (Benadryl)
   C. Change the medication to a phenothiazine
   D. Change the medication to a tricyclic antidepressant
   E. Add phenobarbital
   F. Increase the dose by 50%

Discussion

Different children may require different stimulant doses. A particular child may require a great deal more stimulant than another, since there are large individual differences in blood levels in children of the same body weight with comparable dosages of the same drug. A stimulant should be increased until there is a clinical effect or side effects appear. Diphenhydramine has been suggested by some clinicians as efficacious in treating hyperkinetic children. It is frequently started before the use of stimulants. However, there are not yet any good studies demonstrating its efficacy or comparing it with a stimulant. There is general agreement that the sedatives, such as phenobarbital, are usually contraindicated for hyperkinetic syndrome. Additional agents at such an early point in the treatment would only make the clinical picture more confusing.

Case Continued: The patient's mother later calls and states that although the patient has responded to dextroamphetamine, the presence of anorexia and insomnia has been troublesome.

8. Your alternate choice of drugs at this point would include:
   A. Methylphenidate
   B. Imipramine (Tofranil)
   C. Caffeine, administered in coffee
   D. Phenothiazines
   E. Pemoline

Discussion

Anorexia, insomnia, headaches, stomachaches, nausea, and tearfulness are common with methylphenidate, pemoline, and dextroamphetamine use. However, anorexia and insomnia are often frequent and severe with dextroamphetamine. Since the patient has responded to a stimulant, continuation with methylphenidate or pemoline would be most appropriate at this time. Caffeinated coffee twice a day has been reported to be as effective as methylphenidate in one study. However, preliminary results of a well-controlled study using caffeine tablets failed to substantiate this finding.

Case Continued: After 6 months of treatment, the patient's mother is quite gratified by the results, stating that her son is more easily manageable and is doing much better in school. However, she is concerned about the long-term effects of stimulant drugs.

9. The following can be said of long-term effects of dextroamphetamine and methylphenidate:
   A. Some children develop mild to moderate depressive episodes during the course of treatment
   B. There is some suggestion that suppression of growth may occur with the prolonged use of methylphenidate
   C. There seems to be a predilection for hyperkinetic children who have been medicated with stimulants to become drug abusers

Discussion

There does not seem to be a predilection for hyperkinetic children who have been medicated with stimulants to become drug abusers. There is some suggestion that suppression of growth in height may occur with prolonged use. As a result, a psychostimulant should periodically be tapered in dosage and discontinued to see if it is still necessary.

Answers

1. (E)
2. (A, B, and C)
3. (E)
4. (A)
5. (B, D, and F)
6. (A)
7. (F)
8. (A and E)
9. (A and B)

References

1. Strauss, A. and Lehtinen, L.: *Psychopathology and Education of the Brain Injured Child.* Grune and Stratton, New York, 1947.
2. Sogessel, A. and Amatruda, C.: *Developmental Diagnosis*, second edition. Hans Hœber, New York, p. 248.
3. Clements, S.: *Minimal Brain Dysfunction in Children.* NINDB Monograph No. 3. U.S. Public Health Service, Washington, D.C., 1966.
4. Rutter, M., Lebovic, S., Eisenberg, L., *et al.*: A tri-axial classification of mental disorders of childhood. *Journal of Child Psychology and Psychiatry*, 10: 41–61, 1969.

5. Cantwell, D. P.: *The Hyperactive Child: Diagnosis, Management, Current Research*. Spectrum Publications, New York, 1975.
6. Werry, J.: Developmental hyperactivity. *Pediatric Clinics of North America*, 15(3): 581–599, 1968.
7. Morris, J. and Stewart, N.: A family study of the hyperactive child syndrome. *Biological Psychiatry*, 3: 189–195, 1971.
8. Millichap, J. G. and Fowler, G.: Treatment of minimal brain dysfunction syndrome. *Pediatric Clinics of North America*, 14: 767, 1967.
9. O'Malley, J. and Eisenberg, L.: The hyperkinetic syndrome. *Seminars in Psychiatry*, 5: 95–103, 1973.
10. Conners, C.: Recent drug studies with hyperkinetic children. *Journal of Learning Disabilities*, 4: 476–484, 1971.
11. Wazer, J., *et al.*: Outpatient treatment of hyperactive school children with imipramine. *American Journal of Psychiatry*, 131: 587–591, 1974.
12. Conners, C.: The use of stimulant drugs in enhancing performance learning. In: *Drugs and Cerebral Function* (ed.: W. L. Smith). Charles C Thomas Co., Springfield, IL, 1970.
13. Schnackenberg, R. C.: Caffeine as a substitute for Schedule II stimulants in hyperkinetic children. *American Journal of Psychiatry*, 130: 769–798, 1973.
14. Safer, D., Allen, R., and Barr, E.: Depression of growth in hyperactive children on stimulant drugs. *New England Journal of Medicine*, 287: 217–220, 1972.
15. Katz, S., *et al.*: Clinical pharmacological management of hyperkinetic children. *International Journal of Mental Health*, 4: 157–181, 1975.
16. Barkley, R.: A review of stimulant drug research with hyperactive children. *Journal of Clinical Psychology and Psychiatry*, 18: 137–165, 1977.
17. Cantwell, D. and Carlson, G.: Stimulants. In: *Pediatric Psychopharmacology: The Use of Behavior Modifying Drugs in Children* (ed.: J. S. Werry). Brunner/Mazel, New York, 1980.
18. Anders, T. F. and Ciaranello, R. D.: Pharmacologic treatment of the minimal brain dysfunction syndrome. In: *Psychopharmacology: From Theory to Practice* (eds.: J. D. Barchas, P. A. Berger, R. D. Ciarnello, and G. R. Gershon). Oxford University Press, New York, 1977, p. 425.
19. Aman, M. and Werry, J.: Methylphenidate and diazepam in severe reading retardation. *Journal of the American Academy of Child Psychiatry*, 21(1): 31–37, 1982.
20. Werry, J. and Sprague, R.: Methylphenidate in children: Effects of dosage. *Australian and New Zealand Journal of Psychiatry*, 8: 9–19, 1974.

SECTION VII
IATROGENIC PSYCHOLOGIC DISORDERS

CASE 60: DEPRESSION ASSOCIATED WITH ORAL CONTRACEPTIVES

The patient is a 23-year-old woman who comes to see you complaining of depression. She has no known psychiatric history, but does report having had occasional periods of sadness, lasting several days, during her teenage and early adult years. Her present depression has been more continuous and has been present since she began taking a progestogen-type birth control pill prior to seeing you.

1. Correct statements about depression associated with oral contraceptives include:
   A. Most studies report depression in 50% of women taking oral contraceptives
   B. The depression associated with these drugs is less likely than an endogenous depression to have an associated sleep disorder
   C. Mania is frequently reported with oral-contraceptive use
   D. The depression associated with oral contraceptives is less likely than an endogenous depression to be accompanied by anorexia or weight loss

Discussion

Clinical depression is not often seen in women taking oral contraceptives. The reported incidence is usually approximately 6%. The depression associated with oral-contraceptive use is most frequently an affective change, and does not include vegetative signs such as sleep or appetite disturbance. The most predominant symptoms are pessimism, dissatisfaction, crying, and tension. Mania is infrequently seen.

2. Correct statements about those women most likely to have depressive symptoms while receiving oral contraceptives include:
   A. They are also likely to have depressions following pregnancy
   B. They are also likely to have depressions premenstrually
   C. They are likely to have family histories of depression
   D. All of the above

Discussion

While some physicians feel that oral contraceptives may be useful in alleviating premenstrual tension and depression, a number of women may become seriously depressed with the continued use of these drugs. Women who have a personal or family history of depressive disorder, severe premenstrual tension, or depression during or following pregnancy are those most likely to develop oral-contraceptive-induced depression. It has also been reported that the more strongly progestogenic oral contraceptives cause a greater degree of depression. None of the previous associations has been definitely proven, and most careful investigators agree that the final answer is not in and that individual patients may have biogenetic as well as emotional predispositions toward depression which combine with the physiologic and psychologic effects of the contraceptive to cause the depression. The depression, once present, sometimes disappears as the birth control is continued. Cessation of oral contraceptives may be necessary for the depression to remit.

3. In treating this patient, there is evidence that one should consider using:
   A. Tricyclic antidepressants
   B. Tranylcypromine (Nardil)
   C. L-Tryptophan
   D. All of the above

Discussion

The treatment for depression associated with oral contraceptive use has not definitely worked out. Some physicians employ tricyclic antidepressants in doses similar to those used in endogenous depression. Others add estogenic compounds or use monoamine oxidase inhibitors (MAOIs) such as tranylcypromine. A disturbance in indolamine metabolism has led some investigators to administer pyridoxine or L-tryptophan as a treatment, although the efficency of these treatments is uncertain.

4. The data on the use of L-tryptophan in the treatment of depression indicate that:
   A. L-Tryptophan may be more effective in treating unipolar than bipolar depression
   B. Most patients will have to be treated with 6 to 8 g of L-tryptophan per day before a response is seen
   C. There is conflicting evidence regarding the efficacy of L-tryptophan, with difficulty in replicating studies that show L-tryptophan to be as effective as electroconvulsive therapy (ECT)
   D. All of the above

Discussion

L-Tryptophan has been used in the treatment of depression. The rationale is based on the premise that serotonin is deficient in depression, and that the deficiency is the cause of the depression. Therefore, L-tryptophan, an essential amino acid and a precursor of serotonin, is administered. Several controlled studies have attempted to compare L-tryptophan with antidepressant drugs and ECT, but none has demonstrated conclusively that L-tryptophan is effective. Most studies use between 5 and 10 g of L-tryptophan per day, split into two or three doses.

Answers

1. (B and D)
2. (D)
3. (D)
4. (D)
5. (D)

References

1. Winston, F.: Oral contraceptives, pyridoxine, and depression. *American Journal of Psychiatry*, 130: 1217–1221, 1973.
2. Herrington, R. N., Bruce, A., Johnstone, E. C., and Lader, M. H.: Comparative trial of L-tryptophan and ECT in severe depressive illness. *Lancet*, 2:731–734, 1974.
3. Rausch, J. L., Janowsky, D. S., Risch, S. C., Judd, L. L., and Huey, L. Y.: Hormonal and neurotransmitter hypotheses of premenstrual tension. *Psychopharmacology Bulletin*, 18(4): 25–34, 1982.

CASE 61: TRICYCLIC-ANTIDEPRESSANT-INDUCED CENTRAL ANTICHOLINERGIC SYNDROME

A 68-year-old lady is showing symptoms of chronic depression. Her internist puts her on 150 mg per day of amitriptyline (Elavil). After a period of 10 days, the patient becomes confused. She does not know where she is and she begins to visually hallucinate. She seems to have great difficulty concentrating. She develops hypotension.

1. The confusional episode occurring in this patient is most likely due to:
   A. Cerebral arteriosclerosis
   B. Amitriptyline's side effects on the central nervous system
   C. Activation of latent schizophrenia
   D. Senility
2. The biologic cause of the confusional state is probably:
   A. A central anticholinergic syndrome
   B. Depression of cortical evoked responses
   C. Cortical depression, such as occurs with a barbiturate
   D. Hyperadrenergic stimuli
3. The most reasonable treatment(s) for this patient involve(s):
   A. Supportive medical care
   B. Discontinuation of amitriptyline or reduction in amitriptyline dosage
   C. Serial mental-status examinations

D. All of the above
E. None of the above

Case Continued: After 48 hours of not receiving amitriptyline, the patient is no longer confused. She is, however, still depressed.

4. The most reasonable plan should involve:
   A. Switching to a 150 mg dose of imipramine (Tofranil)
   B. Reinstating amitriptyline at a lower dose, such as 75 mg per day
   C. Beginning a monoamine oxidase inhibitor such as tranylcypromine (Parnate)
   D. None of the above

Discussion

Confusional states in patients over 40 years of age who are receiving tricyclic antidepressants occur with progressive frequency with age and are probably due to the tricyclic antidepressant's central anticholinergic properties. They are usually reversible within 48 hours of drug withdrawal. Physostigmine rapidly clears these states, but probably is less desirable in most cases than conservative management, due to its side effects. The confusional states are probably dose-related, and the reinstitution of tricyclic antidepressant therapy at a lower dose is probably acceptable and indicated. Switching to an equivalent dose of another drug is probably not indicated, since the tricyclic antidepressants generally cross-react in causing confusional states. Trazodone or desipramine may be indicated as alternative agents because of their lack or low frequency of anticholinergic effects. The confusional states caused by tricyclic antidepressants often go unrecognized, or are attributed to senility or other medical conditions.

Answers

1. (B)
2. (A)
3. (D)
4. (B)

References

1. Fann, W. E. and Maddox, G. L.: *Drug Issues in Geropsychiatry*. Williams and Wilkins, Baltimore, 1974.
2. Davis, R. F., Tucker, G. J., Harrow, M., and Detre, T. P.: Confusional episodes and tricyclic antidepressant medication. *American Journal of Psychiatry*, 128: 95–99, 1971.
3. Janowsky, D. S., Davis, J. M., El-Yousef, M. K., and Sekerke, H. J.: Combined anticholinergic agents and atropine-like delirium.. *American Journal of Psychiatry*, 129: 360–361, 1972.
4. Gershon, S. and Newton, R.: Lack of anticholinergic side effects with a new antidepressant trazodone. *Journal of Clinical Psychiatry*, 41: 100, 1980.
5. El-Fakahany, E. and Richelson, E.: Antagonism by antidepressants of muscarinic acetylcholine receptors of human brain. *British Journal of Pharmacology*, 78: 97–102, 1983.
6. Snyder, S. H. and Yamamura, H. T.: Antidepressants and the muscarinic acetylcholine receptor. *Archives of General Psychiatry*, 34: 236–239, 1977.
7. Ordinway, M. V.: Treating tricyclic overdose with physostigmine. *American Journal of Psychiatry*, 135: 1114, 1978.
8. Biggs, J. T., Riesenberg, R. A., and Ziegler, V. E.: Overdosing the tricyclic overdose patient. *American Journal of Psychiatry*, 134: 461–462, 1977.
9. Baldessarini, R. J. and Gelenberg, A. J.: Using physostigmine safely. *American Journal of Psychiatry*, 136: 1608–1609, 1979.

CASE 62: ANTIHYPERTENSIVE-INDUCED DEPRESSION

A 58-year-old man has an history of having had four intermittent major depressive episodes over the past 20 years. He has had no depression for the past 4 months. He has experienced intermittent chest pains, associated with anxiety. The patient visits several physicians and ultimately a diagnosis of angina pectoris is made. The patient is begun on treatment with propranolol 10 mg, q.i.d. for treatment of his angina pectoris.

1. Cardiovascular drugs likely to induce depression include:
   A. Propranolol
   B. Guanethidine
   C. Chlorothiazide diuretics

D. Reserpine
E. A and D
F. A and C

Discussion

Depression is not infrequently induced in individuals given centrally acting catecholamine-depleting or catecholamine-blocking agents. Drugs reported to cause depression include alpha-methyldopa, clonidine, propranolol, and reserpine. Although not proven, it is likely that atenolol, metoprolol, and guanethidine are less likely to cause depression owing to their relative lack of central effects. Similarly, thiazide diuretics do not seem to cause depression. Furthermore, it is important to be aware that hypertension or angina which the above drugs may be used to treat, may themselves precipitate a depressive reaction due to psychologic factors and that such a depression may therefore not be drug induced.

2. Depression, as opposed to lethargy, is most likely to occur in patients treated with catecholamine-depleting agents who have:
   A. A past history of depression
   B. A family history of depression
   C. None of the above
   D. Both of the above
3. Patients receiving glucocorticoids such as prednisone or cortisol are most likely to have a depressive or manic reaction from these medications if they have:
   A. A past history of depression
   B. A family history of depression
   C. None of the above
   D. Both of the above

Discussion

There is evidence that vulnerability to depression following treatment with catecholamine-depleting and -blocking agents and oral contraceptives exists in patients with a past history or a family history of depression. In contrast, the adrenocortical hormones, such as prednisone or cortisol, can cause depression, but in this case affective symptoms are not linked to a history of depression.

Answers

1. (E)
2. (D)
3. (C)

References

1. Bigger, J. T., Kantor, S. J., Glassman, A. H., and Perel, J. M.: Cardiovascular effects of tricyclic antidepressants. In: *Psychopharmacology: A Generation of Progress* (eds.: M. A. Lipton, A. DiMascio, and K. F. Killam). Raven Press, New York, 1978.
2. Risch, S. C., Groom, G., and Janowsky, D. S.: The effects of psychotropic drugs on the cardiovascular system. *Journal of Clinical Psychiatry*, 43: 16–31, 1982.
3. Risch, S. C., Groom, G., and Janowsky, D. S.: Interfaces of psychopharmacology and cardiology: Part II. *Journal of Clinical Psychiatry*, 42: 47–59, 1981.
4. Gaultieri, C. and Powell, S.: Psychoactive drug interactions. *Journal of Clinical Psychiatry*, 39: 720–729, 1978.
5. Alexopoulos, G. S. and Shamoian, C. A.: Tricyclic antidepressants and cardiac patients with pacemakers. *American Journal of Psychiatry*, 139(4): 519–520, 1982.
6. Pariser, S. F., Reynolds, J. C., Falko, J. M., Jones, B. A., and Mencer, D. L.: Arrhythmia induced by a tricyclic antidepressant in a patient with undiagnosed mitral valve prolapse. *American Journal of Psychiatry*, 138(4): 522–523, 1981.
7. Glassman, A. H. and Bigger, J. T.: Cardiovascular effects of therapeutic doses of tricyclic antidepressants: A review. *Archives of General Psychiatry*, 38: 815–820, 1981.

CASE 63: PSYCHOSIS FOLLOWING L-DOPA THERAPY

A 61-year-old oriental married male accountant is referred to you by his neurologist owing to progressive confusion and agitation developing over the previous week. He has had a 3-year history of disabling Parkinson's disease treated with anticholinergic agents. Two weeks previously, he was begun on L-dopa. A psychiatric examination reveals a casually dressed, gray-haired man whose speech is tangential and whose manner is confused. His activity level is heightened, with frequent changes of position in his chair and walking about the room. He shares with the examiner the fact that he has become increasingly involved with business transactions, and believes the Internal Revenue Service recently has put his house under surveillance. He boasts that he has gained heightened sexuality, with increased ability to maintain erection and increased libido.

1. The clinical picture could fit which of the following diagnosis?
   A. Manic–depressive disease, manic type
   B. Hypomanic denial in a patient with a chronic somatic illness
   C. A toxic psychosis with mania secondary to anticholinergic drugs
   D. Central nervous system side effect of L-dopa administration
   E. All of the above

Discussion

The patient described above exhibits multiple features that could support any of the above diagnoses. It would be important to determine whether or not prior affective illness existed in this man, since the acute onset of a first manic episode with no prior history of manic–depressive episodes at the age of 61 is possible but unlikely. Frequently, hypomanic defenses occur in response to serious somatic illnesses. However, in the above case, there appear to be significant organic components, such as confusion, which suggest a toxic etiology. Anticholinergic agents, including trihexyphenidyl (Artane) and benztropine mesylate (Cogentin), as well as tricyclic antidepressants, which have anticholinergic effects, can also produce a toxic psychosis. L-Dopa has been shown to have a wide variety of psychiatric effects, the most common of which is confusion.

2. The most likely diagnosis in this case is:
   A. Manic–depressive illness, manic type
   B. Hypomanic denial in a patient with a chronic somatic illness
   C. A toxic psychosis with mania secondary to anticholinergic drugs
   D. Central-nervous-system side effects of L-dopa

Discussion

The onset of a combination of paranoid ideation, hyperactivity, hypomanic thought content, and confusional elements following L-dopa therapy make the diagnosis of L-dopa-induced psychosis most likely.

3. The most appropriate treatment would be:
   A. Lithium carbonate 300 mg p.o., t.i.d.
   B. Supportive psychotherapy
   C. Resumption of the anticholinergic agent
   D. Decreasing the L-dopa dosage
   E. Electroconvulsive therapy (ECT)

Discussion

The treatment of choice for this patient would be a diminution in the dose of his medication, in the hope that this would limit its psychiatric side effects. If the patient showed continued vulnerability to the central nervous system effects of L-dopa, the L-dopa therapy might have to be abandoned. Reduction of the anticholinergic drug dosage would be indicated. Lithium carbonate would not be indicated as a first line of treatment unless a definitive diagnosis of manic–depressive illness were established. Since the patient presents with very little in the way of a significant mood disturbance or serious retarded depression, ECT would probably not be of value, and might only further confuse the patient.

Case Continued: A further history reveals that there have been no prior episodes of mania or depression in this patient's past. In addition, there have been no significant changes in his drug management, other than the commencement of L-dopa therapy. The working diagnosis becomes an L-dopa-induced psychosis.

4. Behavioral disturbances as a result of L-dopa treatment occur at a frequency of:
   A. 1%
   B. 5%
   C. 20%
   D. 75%
   E. 90%

Discussion

The average incidence of psychiatric side effects associated with L-dopa treatment is approximately 20%, with a reported range of 10% to 50%. Variability in the incidence of psychiatric side effects depends on patient selection, as well as on the researchers' sensitivity to such effects.

5. Other groups of symptoms which occur more commonly than psychiatric problems in patients treated with L-dopa are:
   A. Gastrointestinal effects
   B. Genitourinary effects
   C. Movement disorders
   D. Cardiovascular effects
   E. Visual disturbances

Discussion

Abnormal movements (e.g., dyskinesias) and gastrointestinal side effects are the two groups of side effects which occur more commonly than psychiatric side effects with the use of L-dopa in Parkinson's disease patients.

6. L-Dopa is administered instead of dopamine in the treatment of parkinsonism because:
   A. Dopamine causes gastrointestinal disturbances
   B. Dopamine causes hypertensive crises
   C. Dopamine is more rapidly excreted

D. Dopamine competes with norepinephrine in crossing the blood–brain barrier
E. Dopamine does not cross the blood–brain barrier

7. L-Dopa is the amino acid precursor of:
   A. Epinephrine
   B. Norepinephrine
   C. Dopamine
   D. All of the above
   E. None of the above

Discussion

Neither norepinephrine nor dopamine can cross the blood–brain barrier. The epinephrine, norepinephrine, and dopamine precursor L-dopa can penetrate the barrier and therefore can affect central-nervous-system function.

8. The rationale for the use of L-dopa is that a dopamine deficiency exists in certain areas of the brain in parkinson's disease patients. The basic concept in the use of L-dopa is that it represents:
   A. A substitute for dopamine
   B. A blocking agent of dopamine
   C. A precursor of dopamine
   D. An antagonist of dopamine
   E. A false transmitter

Discussion

The underlying rationale for using L-dopa is that this amino acid is a precursor of dopamine in the brain, especially in the area of the presumed dopamine deficiency.

9. Match the following words with the appropriate descriptive phrase:
   A. Precursor substance
   B. Antagonist
   C. False transmitter

(1) Chemical substance capable of occupying an identical site at the neurosynapse, but with a different activity
(2) Agent having an opposite effect
(3) A compound which will precede the synthesis of the desired compound in a metabolic pathway

10. The most commonly reported psychiatric side effect of L-dopa is:
    A. Confusion and disorientation
    B. Hypomania
    C. Paranoia
    D. Depression

Discussion

Confusion, disorientation, and sometimes delirium have been observed in studies of the side effects of L-dopa. The most commonly reported side effect of this drug is therefore an organic brain syndrome. However, other psychiatric disturbances, including hypomania, paranoia, and depression have been observed with L-dopa therapy.

11. In the psychosis secondary to L-dopa administration, the clinical picture may consist of:
    A. Paranoid delusions
    B. Visual and olfactory hallucinations
    C. A heightened activity level
    D. All of the above
    E. None of the above

Discussion

Wide variations exist in the percentage of patients who develop psychotic symptoms while receiving L-dopa depending on the type of the patient group selected. Patients in a lower age group without pre-existing confusional states have a much smaller chance of developing psychotic symptoms. Patients with a past history of schizophrenia demonstrate a greater risk of developing psychotic symptoms. The psychotic symptoms are often characterized by paranoia, hyperactivity, visual hallucinations, and even olfactory hallucinations, such as are often seen in toxic conditions. The use of L-dopa in the treatment of parkinsonism has now become established. L-Dopa is an amino acid precursor of the catecholamines dopamine, and norepinephrine. These neurotransmitters are intimately related to various types of cerebral functions, and therefore patients receiving L-dopa therapy must be carefully observed for changes in behavior, mood disturbances, and thinking disorders. Although it has been stated by some that most parkinsonian patients experience an improvement in mood on L-dopa episodes of severe depression have been reported as a consequence of this treatment. When elevation of mood occurs, it may be related to the central nervous system effects of L-dopa or to the patient's anticipated and grateful sense of well-being secondary to an improvement in his neurological status. Although the characteristic behavioral manifestations of L-dopa toxicity include confusion and delirium, depression, delusions, hypomania, and heightened sexuality, secondary depression with L-dopa therapy may result from a patient's reaction to treatment failure. Some preliminary studies have attempted to use L-dopa in the treatment of primary psychogenic impotence. Results from these studies have varied. It is important to note that many patients with impotence suffer from a primary depression and that this depression may be exacerbated by the use of L-dopa. The possibility of enhanced learning and increased memory in depressed patients following L-dopa administration has been suggested.

Answers

1. (E)
2. (D)
3. (D)
4. (C)
5. (A and C)
6. (E)
7. (D)
8. (C)
9. (A-3, B-2, C-1)
10. (A)
11. (D)

References

1. Murphy, D. L., Brodie, H. K. H., Goodwin, F. K., and Bunney, W. E., Jr.: L-Dopa: Regular induction of hypomania in bipolar manic–depressive patients. *Nature*, 229: 135, 1971.

2. Goodwin, F. K.: Behavioral effects of L-dopa in man. *Seminars in Psychiatry*, 3(4): 477–492, 1971.
3. Barbeau, A.: Long-term side effects of levodopa. *Lancet*, 1: 395, 1971.
4. McDowell, F., *et al.*: Treatment of Parkinson's syndrome with L-dihydroxyphenylalanine (levodopa). *Annals of Internal Medicine*, 72: 29, 1970.
5. Goodwin, F. K., *et al.*: L-Dopa, catecholamines and behavior: A clinical and biochemical study in the depressed patient. *Biological Psychiatry*, 2: 341, 1970.
6. Jenkins, R. B. and Groh, R. H.: Mental symptoms in parkinsonian patients treated with L-dopa. *Lancet*, 2: 177, 1970
7. Knopp, W.: Psychiatric changes in patients treated with levodopa: I. Clinical experiment. *Neurology*, 20: 23, 1970.
8. Meier, N. J. and Martin, W. E.: Intellectual changes associated with levodopa therapy. *Journal of the American Medical Association*, 213: 465, 1970.
9. Mindham, R. H. S.: Psychiatric symptoms in parkinsonism. *Journal of Neurological and Neurosurgical Psychiatry*, 33: 188, 1970.
10. O'Brien, C. T., DiGiacomo, J. N., Fahn, S., and Schwartz, G. A.: Mental effects of high dosage levodopa. *Archives of General Psychiatry*, 24: 61–64, 1971.
11. Selesia, G. G. and Barr, A. N.: Psychosis and other psychiatric manifestations of levodopa therapy. *Archives of Neurology*, 23: 193, 1970.
12. Charington, M.: Parkinsonism, L-dopa and mental depression. *Journal of the American Geriatric Society*, 18: 513, 1970.
13. Creese, I. and Leff, S.: Dopamine receptors: A classification. *Journal of Clinical Psychopharmacology*, 2: 329–335, 1982.
14. Smith, J. M.: Abuse of antiparkinsonian drugs: A review of the literature. *Journal of Clinical Psychiatry*, 41: 351–354, 1980.
15. Flaherty, J. A.: Psychiatric complications of medical drugs. *Journal of Family Practice*, 9(2): 243–251, 1979.
16. Danielson, D. A., Porter, J. B., Lawson, D. H., Soubrie, C., and Jick, H.: Drug-associated psychiatric disturbances in medical inpatients. *Psychopharmacology*, 74: 1055–108, 1981.

CASE 64: CENTRAL ANTICHOLINERGIC SYNDROME FOLLOWING INGESTION OF AN OVER-THE-COUNTER SLEEPING PREPARATION

A 36-year-old female patient is brought to the emergency room of the hospital because 12 hours earlier she had taken an undetermined number of sleeping pills in a suicide attempt. The patient presents as confused, disoriented, and hallucinating. She stays under the bedcovers and constantly thrashes around in bed. She expresses paranoid ideation, insisting that a woman friend is trying to kill her. She constantly sees herself being placed in a casket. Her vital signs are: a blood pressure of 148/80 mm Hg, pulse of 95, respiration of 18, pupils fixed and dilated, skin hot and dry, and an oral temperature of 98.6°F. Her mucous membranes are very dry.

1. The most likely diagnosis is:
   A. Schizophrenia, paranoid type
   B. Paranoid state
   C. Manic-depressive illness
   D. Organic brain syndrome with psychosis
2. The clinical signs and symptoms that would support a diagnosis of organic brain syndrome with psychosis include:
   A. Dilated pupils
   B. Visual hallucinations
   C. Rapidity of onset
   D. Paranoid ideation

Discussion

A definitive history of overdosing on sleeping tablets in a suicide attempt preceding arrival in the emergency room would suggest that a toxic reaction has occurred. Dilation of pupils and the presence of visual hallucinations would likewise suggest a toxic agent. Paranoid ideation as such would be consistent with any of a number of diagnoses, and therefore would not be diagnostically specific in this case. It is often difficult to get a clear psychiatric history or to differentiate functional from organic diagnoses in severely agitated patients. Visual hallucinations also suggest toxic contributions to the presenting symptoms.

Case Continued: The patient's friend states that she had ingested 50 tablets of a common over-the-counter sleep preparation.

3. The drug producing the syndrome being evaluated is quite likely to be:
   A. Scopolamine
   B. Methapyrilene hydrochloride

C. Pyridoxine hydrochloride
D. Salicylamide

Discussion

There has been an increasing incidence of patients presenting with a clinical picture similar to that of an acute schizophrenic reaction, caused by ingesting over-the-counter sleeping pills. These agents contain a number of additional chemicals such as methapyrilene, salicylamide, and vitamin preparations. However, the active psychotoxic ingredient is usually scopolamine or a centrally-acting anticholinergic agent.

4. In the absence of a history of taking over-the-counter sleeping agents, a confirmative diagnosis could be obtained through:
   A. Thin-layer chromatography of the urine
   B. Electroencephalography
   C. Neurological examination
   D. Methacholine injection

Discussion

To identify a case of anticholinergic toxicity, a hypodermic injection of 10 to 30 mg methacholine may be of value. If the typical cutaneous flush, salivation, sweating, lacrimation, intestinal hyperactivity, and other signs of cholinergic activation do not occur, anticholinergic intoxication is a certainty because anticholinergic agents antagonize the muscarinic actions of methacholine. Since only 1% of scopolamine is excreted in the urine, an analysis of the patient's urine by thin-layer chromatography might be positive for additional agents found in over-the-counter sleeping pills, including methapyrilene and salicylamide, but would not be positive for scopolamine.

5. The drug of choice for a scopolamine-induced toxic psychosis is:
   A. Chlorpromazine (Thorazine)
   B. Diazepam (Valium)
   C. Physostigmine (Antilirium)
   D. Neostigmine (Prostigmin)

Discussion

Physostigmine is an initial dose of 1 to 2 mg i.m. is the drug of choice in treating central anticholinergic symptoms. Its action occurs within 15 to 20 minutes, and complete restoration of the patient's normal mental processes will usually occur. Repeated dosages of physostigmine are indicated. In some patients, the response to physostigmine is incomplete. In some studies it is suggested that if physostigmine is not given until 12 to 18 hours after ingestion of an anticholinergic agent, there may be failure to obtain improvement with this drug.

Case Continued: Despite an immediate clearing of the sensorium following an initial injection of physostigmine, the patient's condition later shows a return of symptoms, with increased confusion, restlessness, and a return of pupillary dilatation.

6. The reason for this relapse is:
   A. A mistaken diagnosis
   B. Increasing serum level of the toxin, due to further absorption
   C. Rapid metabolism of physostigmine
   D. None of the above

Discussion

Although there may be a continued presence of scopolamine, physostigmine is short acting and therefore may require additional dosage at intervals of 45 to 60 minutes, depending on the clinical status of the patient.

Answers

1. (D)
2. (A, B, and C)
3. (A)
4. (D)
5. (C)
6. (C)

References

1. Bernstein, S. and Leff, R.: Toxic psychosis from sleeping medicines containing scopolamine. *New England Journal of Medicine*, 277: 638–639, 1967.
2. Smith, J. M.: Abuse of antiparkinsonian drugs: A review of the literature. *Journal of Clinical Psychiatry*, 41: 351–354, 1980.
3. Crowell, E. B. and Ketchum, J. S.: Treatment of scopolamine-induced delirium with physostigmine. *Clinical Pharmacology and Therapeutics*, 8: 409–414, 1967.
4. Ulman, K. C. and Groh, R. H.: Identification and treatment of acute psychotic state secondary to the use of over-the-counter sleep preparations. *American Journal of Psychiatry*, 128(10): 1244–1248, 1972.
5. Baldessarini, R. J. and Gelenberg, A. J.: Using physostigmine safely. *American Journal of Psychiatry*, 136: 1608–1609, 1979.

INDEX

ACTH. *See* Adrenocorticotropic hormone
ADD. *See* Attention deficit disorder
Adrenocorticotropic hormone (ACTH), 109
Affective disorders, 53–146
  depression, 53–58. *See also* Antidepressants
    bipolar, 78–99, 105–108, 123–126, 138–144
    in elderly, 115–123
    pseudo-dementia and, 61–67
    resistant, 67–72
    unipolar, 53–61, 85, 93
  electroconvulsive therapy for, 108–113
  guanethidine-imipramine interactions and, 126–128
  in hemodialysis patient, 133–137
  insomnia and, 162
  monoamine oxidase inhibitor-tricyclic antidepressant therapy in, 128–133
  premenstrual syndrome and, 144–146
  premenstrual tension and, 113–115
  schizophreniform disorder, 99–104
Agranulocytosis, 16
Akathisias, 31
Alcohol, barbiturates and, 178, 179
Alcoholism, 54
  drug treatment of, 184–191
  insomnia and, 162
  lithium and, 105
  propranolol and, 161
  Wernicke-Korsakoff syndrome and, 194–197
  withdrawal and, 184–187
Allergic reactions to antidepressants, 70, 71
Alpha-methyldopa, 46, 240
Alprazolam (Xanax), 152
Amatadine (Symmetrel), 31
Amitriptyline (Elavil), 54, 73, 74
Amnesia, anterograde, 111
Amoxapine, 68, 69, 71, 74, 77
Anticholinergic effects, 15, 16
  of antidepressants, 74
Anticonvulsants, 211
Antidepressants, 50, 54–61, 236
  cancer pain and, 211
  confusion caused by, 237–239
  dementia and, 64–66
  electroconvulsive therapy compared to, 112
  the elderly and, 117–123
  in hemodialysis patient, 133–137
  hyperkinetic children and, 229
  imipramine, 54–61, 73
  lithium as, 98, 99
  lithium used with, 86, 87, 92–94
  monoamine oxidase inhibitors combined with, 128–132
  new, 54, 73

Antidepressants, (*continued*)
panic attacks and, 152
premenstrual tension and, 114
side effects of, 55, 68–75, 120
Antilirium (physostigmine), 31, 250, 251
Antimanic drugs
carbamazepine, 95–98
lithium, 78–98, 105–108
Antinoradrenergic effects, 15, 16
Antipsychotic drugs, 1-4, 11–40
indications for specific, 40–43
maintenance therapy, 17–24, 32–37
new, 75–78
organic brain syndrome and, 171, 172
relapse-sensitive patient and, 51, 52
side effects of, 13–17, 29–40
extrapyramidal symptoms, 16, 29–32
tardive dyskinesia, 3, 32–40, 43–47
Anxiety
"anticipatory," 154
chronic, 188
situational, 147–151
treatment of, 147–151, 155–161
antianxiety agents, 155–158
propranolol, 158–161
Anxiety attacks, 53, 54, 157
Artane (trihexyphenidyl), 31, 242
Atenolol, 240
Attention deficit disorder (ADD), 227, 228

Barbiturates, 178–183, 214, 215
alcohol and, 178, 179
Bedwetting, 216–221
Benadryl (diphenhydramine), 31, 229, 231
Benzodiazepines, 45, 137, 149, 150, 155–158
side effects of, 157, 158
withdrawal from 192, 193
Benztropine mesylate (Cogentin), 16, 31, 34, 35, 46, 242
Beta-receptors, 159
Bipolar illness. *See* Depression, bipolar
Birth control pills, depression and, 234–237, 240
Bupropion, 73
Butaperazine, 42
Butyrophenone, 23, 46

Cancer pain, 207–212
Carbamazepine, 95–98
Central anticholinergic syndrome, 248–252
Central nervous system, 223
lithium's effect on, 88
propranolol and, 159, 160
Childhood disorders, 216–233
enuresis, 216–221
Gilles de la Tourette syndrome, 221–226
hyperactivity, 226–233
Chlordiazepoxide (Librium), 54, 148–150, 154, 155
alcohol withdrawal and, 185
for confusion, 173, 174
Chlorpromazine, 16, 42, 54, 139, 140
Cholestatic hepatic effects, 16
Clonidine, 39, 199, 240
Cogentin (benztropine mesylate), 16, 31, 34, 35, 46, 242
Confusion
antidepressants and, 237–239
electroconvulsive therapy and, 111
in an elderly man, 173, 174
treatment of, 169–172
Corticosteroids, 211
Cortisol, 241

Cortisone, 109
Cylert (pemoline), 229, 230

Dalmane (flurazepam), 167
Darvon-N (propoxyphene napsylate), 199
Deanol, 45
Dementia versus pseudo-dementia, 61–67
Depression, 53–78
  alcoholism and, 189
  antihypertensive-induced, 239–241
  bipolar, 78–99
    carbamazepine, 95–98
    in elderly, 123–126, 138–144
    lithium, 78–99, 105–108
    maintenance drug therapy, 83–95
  in elderly, 115–123
  oral contraceptives and, 234–237, 240
  pseudo-dementia and, 61–67
  reserpine-induced, 50
  resistant, 67–72
  unipolar, 53–61, 85, 93
Desipramine (Norpramin), 64, 73–76, 152, 153, 238
Desoxyn (dextroamphetamine), 229, 230
Dexamethasone, 211
Dextroamphetamine (Desoxyn), 229, 230
Diazepam (Valium), 39, 88, 148, 149, 153–156
  for confusion, 173, 174
  dependence on, 175–177
  withdrawal from, 191–194
Dilantin (diphenylhydantoin), 185
Diphenhydramine (Benadryl), 31, 229, 231
Diphenylhydantoin (Dilantin), 185
Disulfiram, 187
Diuretics
  alcoholic withdrawal and, 185
  lithium and, 141, 142
Dopamine, 244, 245
Dopamine blockade, 15, 16, 27
L-Dopa therapy, psychosis and, 242–248
Doxepin, 74
Drug abuse, 175–215. *See also* Alcoholism
  diazepam dependence, 175–177
  diazepam withdrawal, 191–194
  heroin detoxification and, 197–201
  insomnia and, 162, 167
  lysergic acid diethylamide (LSD) reaction and, 212, 213
  methadone maintenance therapy and, 201–207
  propranolol, 161
  sedative–hypnotic detoxification and, 213–214
  sedative–hypnotic overdose, 177–184
Drugs. *See also specific drugs*
  antianxiety, 147–150, 155–158
  antidepressant, 50, 54–61
    dementia, 64–66
    elderly and, 117–123
    imipramine, 54–61, 73
    lithium used with, 86, 87, 92–94
    new, 54, 75–78
    side effects, 55, 68–75, 120
  antimanic
    carbamazepine, 95–98
    lithum, 78–98, 105–108
  antipsychotic, 1–4, 11–40
    indications for specific, 40–43
    maintenance therapy, 17–24, 32–37
    relapse-sensitive patients and, 51, 52
    side effects, 24–40, 43–47

Drugs, (*continued*)
chronic pain and, 207–212
genetically linked effectiveness of, 58
Dystonias, 31

ECT. *See* Electroconvulsive therapy
Elavil (amitriptyline), 54, 73, 74
Elderly, the
affective disorders in, 115–123
antidepressants for, 117–123
confusion in, 173, 174
depression in, 115–123
bipolar, 123–126, 138–144
electroconvulsive therapy for, 108–113, 116, 117
lithium for, 140–143
mania in, 123–126, 138–144
organic brain syndrome in, 173, 174
tardive dyskinesia in, 43–47
Electroconvulsive therapy (ECT), 50, 54, 66, 243
complications in, 111
in elderly patients, 108–113, 116, 117
Electroencephalographic (EEG) findings, 223
Enuresis, treatment of, 216–221
Ephedrine, 16
Epinephrine, 245
Eutonyl (pargyline), 129
Extrapyramidal symptoms, 16, 29–32

Flagyl (metronidazole), 189
Fluphenazine, 42
Fluphenazine decanoate, 5
Fluphenazine enanthate, 4–6, 11
Flurazepam (Dalmane), 167
Furosemide, 185

Gilles de la Tourette syndrome, 221–226
haloperidol and, 224, 225
Glutethimide, 137
Goiter formation, 88
Guanethidine (Ismelin), 240
imipramine's interaction with, 126–128

Haldol (haloperidol), 7–9, 40, 42, 96, 140
for confusion, 174
Gilles de la Tourette syndrome and, 224, 225
substitute for, 16
Heroin detoxification, 197–201
Hyperkinetic child syndrome, 226–233
Hypertension, 160
Hypotension, 15, 16
antidepressants and, 70–73

Imipramine (Tofranil), 54–61, 73, 152
bedwetting and, 218–220
guanethidine's interaction with, 126–128
Insomnia
chronic, 165–168
evaluation of, 161–165
treatment of, 161–168
Ismelin (guanethidine), 240
imipramine's interaction with, 126–128
Isoproterenol, beta-receptors and, 159

Jaundice, 16

Kemadrine (procyclidine), 31
Korsakoff's syndrome. *See* Werknicke–Korsakoff syndrome

Librium (chlordiazepoxide), 54, 148–150, 154, 155
  alcohol withdrawal and, 185
  for confusion, 173, 174
Lithium, 78–99, 105–108
  alcoholism and, 105
  as antidepressant, 98, 99
  antidepressants used with, 86, 87, 92–94
  diuretics and, 141, 142
  the elderly and, 140–143
  hyperkinetic children and, 229
  maintenance drug therapy and, 83–95
  premenstrual tension and, 114, 145
  renal failure and, 136
  schizophreniform disorder and, 103
  side effects of, 81, 87–89
Lithium carbonate, 45
LSD (lysergic acid diethylamide), 189, 212, 213

Mania, 78–99. *See also* Depression, bipolar; Lithium
  acute, diagnosis and treatment of, 104–106
  carbamazepine and, 95–98
  compared with schizophreniform disorder, 101
  in the elderly, 123–126, 138–144
  maintenance drug therapy and, 83–95
MAOIs. *See* Monoamine oxidase inhibitors
Maprotiline, 74, 77
MBD. *See* Minimal brain dysfunction
Megavitamin therapy, 186
Methacholine, 250
Methadone, 198, 199
  maintenance therapy, 201–207
Methapyrilene, 250
Methaqualone (Quaalude), 214
Methylphenidate (Ritalin), 228–231
Metoprolol, 88, 240
Metronidazole (Flagyl), 189
Minimal brain dysfunction (MBD), 227, 228
Monoamine oxidase inhibitors (MAOIs), 54, 70, 71, 73, 86, 87, 93, 94, 129–132, 236
  panic attacks and, 152

Nardil (phenelzine), 70, 71, 73, 94, 129, 152
Neurosis (neurotic disorders), 147–168
  anxiety, 155–161
    situational, 147–151
    treatment, 147–151, 155–161
  insomnia, 161–168
  panic attacks, 151–154
Nocturnal myoclonus (restless leg syndrome), 162, 163
Nomifensine, 73
Norepinephrine, 245
Norpramin (desipramine), 64, 73–76, 152, 153, 238
Nortriptyline, 64, 66

Older patients. *See* Elderly, the
Oral contraceptives, 114
  depression and, 234–237, 240
Organic brain syndrome, 169–174
  in an elderly man, 173, 174
  treatment of, 169–172

Pain
  acute versus chronic, 208
  in terminally ill patients, 207–212
Panic attacks, 151–154
Paraldehyde, 185
Pargyline (Eutonyl), 129
Patient–therapist–drug relationship, 21, 22

Phenothiazines, 211
Pemoline (Cylert), 229, 230
Pentobarbital, 178–183
Perphenazine, 1, 2, 10, 11, 42
Phencyclidine (PCP), 213
Phenelzine (Nardil), 70, 71, 73, 94, 129, 152
Phenothiazine, 46, 213
  substitutes for, 23
Phlebitis, 157
Physostigmine (Antilirium), 31, 250, 251
Polyuria, 88
Prednisone, 241
Premenstrual syndrome, 144–146
Premenstrual tension, 113–115
Procyclidine (Kemadrin), 31
Propoxyphene napsylate (Darvon-N), 199
Propranolol, 39, 45, 81, 88, 158–161, 240
Protriptyline, 64, 74
Pseudo-dementia versus dementia, 61–67
Psychosis
  L-dopa therapy and, 242–248
  propranolol and, 161
  rapid tranquilization of, 6–10
  tardive, 38
Pyridoxine, 236

Quaalude (methaqualone), 214

Rapid-eye-movement (REM) sleep, 166
Renal failure, antidepressants and, 133–137
Reserpine, 45–50, 109, 240
  side effects of, 50
  in tardive dyskinesia, 45, 46
Restless leg syndrome (nocturnal myoclonus), 162, 163
Ritalin (methylphenidate), 228–231

Salicylamide, 250
Schizophrenia, 1–52
  acute, 1–4, 6–10, 102
  antipsychotic drugs in, 1–4, 11–40
    indications for specific, 40–43
    maintenance therapy, 17–24, 32–37
    relapse-sensitive patient, 51, 52
    side effects, 13–17, 24–40, 43–47
  chronic, 10–13, 19, 20, 24–28, 47–50, 112
  electroconvulsive therapy and, 112
  extrapyramidal symptoms and, 16, 29–32
  fluphenazine enanthate in, 4–6
  "good-prognosis." *See* Schizophreniform disorder
  patient–therapist–drug relationship in, 21, 22
  rapid tranquilization of, 6–10
  reserpine in, 45–50
  symptoms of, 53
  tardive dyskinesia and, 3, 24–28, 32–40
    in elderly patient, 43–47
Schizophreniform disorder, 99–104
Scopolamine, 163, 164, 213, 250, 251
Seconal (secobarbital), 165–168, 214
Sedation, antidepressants and, 71, 73
Sedative–hypnotic detoxification, 213–215
Sedative–hypnotic overdose, 177–184
Sedatives, 171
Seizures, 180
  alcohol withdrawal, 185, 186
Sleep apnea, 163, 167

Sleep disorders. *See* Insomnia
Sleeping tablets, central
anticholinergic syndrome and, 248–252
Somnolence, 15, 16
Spironolactone, 114
Stelazine (trifluoperazine), 34
Suicide, 188
Surgery, organic brain syndrome and, 170
Symmetrel (amatadine), 31

Tardive dyskinesia, 3, 24–28, 32–40
antidepressants and, 77
antipsychotic drug maintenance and, 32–37
in elderly patient, 43–47
treatment of, 38, 39
Tardive psychosis, 38
Tetrabenazine, 46
Thiamine, 186
Wernicke–Korsakoff syndrome and, 195, 197
Thioridazine, 40–42, 139, 140
Thiothixene, 42
Thioxanthene, 23
Thyroid, lithium's effect on, 87, 88
Thyrotoxicosis, 160
Tofranil (imipramine), 54–61, 73, 152
bedwetting and, 218–220
guanethidine's interaction with, 126–128
Tranquilizers, 54, 112, 139, 140
alcoholic rehabilitation and, 187, 188
anxiety and, 147, 148
renal failure and, 135, 136
Tranylcypromine, 73, 129
Trazodone, 73, 76, 238
Tricyclic-antidepressant-induced central anticholinergic syndrome, 237–239
Trifluoperazine (Stelazine), 34, 42
Trihexyphenidyl (Artane), 31, 46, 242
Trimipramine, 93
L-Tryptophan, 166, 236

Valium (diazepam), 88, 148, 149, 153–156
Vomiting, sedative–hypnotic overdose and, 179

Wernicke–Korsakoff syndrome, 194–197

Xanax (alprazolam), 152